HEART ATTACK

The Family Response
at Home and in the Hospital

**SPEEDLING, Edward J. Heart attack: the family response at home
and in the hospital.** Tavistock (dist. by Methuen), 1982. 184p
index 82-650. 18.95 ISBN 0-422-77790-0; 9.95 pa ISBN 0-422-
77800-1. CIP

Speedling provides an understanding and a generalized perspective on what
happens to a family when one of its members suffers a heart attack. As
assistant director of support services at Mount Sinai Hospital in New York
City, Speedling developed a research program that closely followed what
happened to eight families after a member of the immediate family suffered a heart attack. The study began when the patient was placed in the
intensive care unit. Both in the medical wards and at home, attempts were
made to determine how the effects of these environments, the stress of
illness, and the family's understanding of the situation affected their readiness to assume responsibility for care of the ill family member at home. The
author has written a clear, understandable, and well-organized account of
what happens to families in the midst of this type of crisis. The book
identifies most of the key issues that need to be understood by health-care
providers and families to effectively work through these events. This book
provides a framework for understanding the feelings and experiences of
families and demonstrates how to use families in the therapeutic process to

improve the status of the patient and the coping ability of the family.
Strongly recommended for all levels of health professionals and providers
involved with cardiac patients and also for lay people who have a family
member afflicted with heart disease.

To Eileen

HEART ATTACK

The Family Response at Home
and in the Hospital

Edward J. Speedling

Tavistock Publications

NEW YORK and LONDON

First published in 1982 by
Tavistock Publications
in association with Methuen, Inc.
733, Third Avenue, New York, NY 10017
and Tavistock Publications Ltd
11, New Fetter Lane, London EC4P 4EE

© 1982 Edward J. Speedling

Printed in the United States of America

Library of Congress Cataloguing in Publication Data
Speedling, Edward, 1942–
  Heart attack.

  Bibliography: p.
  Includes indexes.
  1. Heart—Infarction—Psychological aspects.
2. Heart—Infarction—Social aspects. 3. Heart—
Infarction—Patients—Family relationships. I. Title.
[DNLM: 1. Coronary disease—Psychology. 2. Family.
WG 300 S742h]
RC685.I6S687   362.8'2   82-650
ISBN 0-422-77790-0   AACR2
ISBN 0-422-77800-1 (pbk.)

British Library Cataloguing in Publication Data
Speedling, Edward
  Heart attack: the family response at home and in
  the hospital.
  1. Cardiovascular patient—Family relationships
  I. Title
  362.8'2'0973   RC682

  ISBN 0-422-77790-0
  ISBN 0-422-77800-1 Pbk

Contents

Preface

One of the more significant requirements of social systems is the ability to adapt to change. Each year hundreds of thousands of families face the unenviable challenge of a heart attack. The initial shock of the event, which can occur with little warning, often sends waves of paralyzing fear throughout the family. Even after the heart itself has been mended, the family's social fabric, its emotional bond, may remain rent. It is to learn more about how family systems adapt to a situation that consists of acute, life-threatening, and chronic dimensions that this study was undertaken.

By closely following what happened to eight families after heart attacks struck we were able to identify the problems that were experienced, and the processes by which family members, individually and collectively, attempted to overcome them. Data was collected by means of in depth interviewing of patients, family members, and medical and nursing staff, and by participant observation in the hospital and in the patients' homes.

The study was initiated in the Intensive Care Unit of the hospital where the patients were treated. Here and in the medical wards we attempted to ascertain the impact of the hospital environment on patients' and families' definitions of the situation and on their readiness to assume responsibility for care at home. Inside the subjects' homes we were able to observe interactional processes that typified different stages of the home-based recovery. Moreover, based on an analysis of each family's internal organization, we have identified an association between styles of coping and adaptation, and characteristics of family structure and value climate.

The study could not have been undertaken, much less

completed, without the active cooperation of the families who at a time of great strain allowed me to enter their private domains. I can only hope that this work justifies the trust they placed in me. This is their book, and I acknowledge the debt of gratitude I and whoever profitably reads this book owe to them. I also want to express my sincere appreciation to the doctors, nurses, and administrators of Group Hospital for being fully cooperative during the course of the time I spent with them.

Support for this project was provided by a grant from the Commonwealth Fund to the Department of Community Medicine, Mt Sinai School of Medicine of the City University of New York where I held a research fellowship. My colleagues both at Mt Sinai and the Graduate Center of the City University of New York provided invaluable assistance. I am particularly grateful to Emily Mumford, Sam Bloom, Arnold Simmel, and Gerald Handel, whose patience and guidance went beyond what I had a right to expect.

Finally, my wife Eileen provided me with a constant source of support and encouragement. Her willingness to spend endless hours discussing the study with me, her insight into human behavior, and her companionship were vital to my ability to sustain the effort required to complete this work.

I

Beginnings

In this book we shall see how the lives of eight families were affected by heart attacks to the husband–fathers. The families are ordinary ones; they lived the kind of lives that are typical for members of the lower middle class. They are stable families, not without problems, but with the inner resources and social supports necessary for managing relationships among their members and with the larger society. Through hard work and saving they lived comfortably in neat houses or apartments and took a real pride in the security their efforts had achieved.

While each stage of life is dynamic, the families we shall be discussing were, in their development, at a point of considerable change. This was a time of children being on their own, of retirement plans, of relocating, and of increased leisure. It is also a time when illness, far from being a sometimes thing, occurs with enough regularity that it must be managed and integrated into one's life.

The study on which this book is based followed events in these lives from the point where treatment of the illness began, the Intensive Care Unit of Group Hospital, to the time when the participants were looking forward to resuming significant work and family roles, about three or four months after the crisis began.

Each of the families received its medical care from the same source: a prepaid group practice. For the most part, they were long-time members of Medical Group, which provided comprehensive primary care and which had its own hospital where the men received medical care for their heart attacks.

The Beginning of the Crisis

Today people stricken with heart attacks are supported by an impressive amount of medical assistance. The modern hospital provides skilled personnel, sophisticated equipment, and effective medications, all of which enhance the patient's chances for survival and ultimate return to the community. Immediately upon admission to the hospital, the heart attack victim is the focal point of a coordinated effort by man and machine.

The beginning of treatment, which occurs once the heart attack victim is within the boundaries of the medical care system, is not the beginning of the personal crisis. In fact admission into the coronary care unit marks the end of a period that is exceedingly difficult for the family to manage. The victim and his loved ones first have to determine the significance of the symptoms being experienced, decide upon a course of action, and finally, under very difficult circumstances, take some decisive action. Initial concern about the pain and the sickness intensifies when it does not respond to the usual remedies for muscle aches, indigestion, heartburn, and whatever else might relieve the dull pressure against the chest, or the sharp stabs in the back or arms. There may be tension at home when, after deciding that the present symptoms are unusually serious, the sufferer and his spouse do not agree on what to do next. When a decision to seek medical help is finally made, there may be uncertainty over whom to call or where to go. This occurs particularly in the evening or at other times outside physicians' office hours. Deciding whether to call an ambulance or drive to the hospital may generate conflict among the family members, as may deciding who will do the driving. By the time the patient is admitted into the Coronary Care Unit, he and his family will very likely have been through a complex and harrowing experience. All are also likely to be exhausted from the preceding hours, even days, of worried indecision and fretful activity.

The experience of Mr and Mrs Polski exemplifies the complexity of the early, pre-hospital phase of crisis. It started on a Saturday morning with a sharp pain while he was hard at work building an extension to the couple's home in the country. Assuming that he had developed a chest cold, he disregarded Mrs Polski's suggestion to rest and continued to work vigorously at his project. Contrary to past experience, working on this particular occasion did not relieve the symptoms but made him feel worse. By afternoon he was forced to lie down, and by nightfall he could not move either arm without intense, crushing pain. He sat up all night. Pain prevented him from sleeping or even lying down. The couple were sixty miles from their family physician. There was a volunteer ambulance corps in the town; in fact, the couple had made contributions to it. Yet although they thought of calling the ambulance, they did not, hoping "it would pass." By Sunday morning – hours after the attack – Mr Polski felt some relief from the pain, enough so he could drive. Over the objections of his wife, who wanted to drive, he took the wheel for the sixty-mile trip to his physician's office.

But he did not drive directly there. Instead, the couple went home to wait until the start of their physician's office hours on Monday morning. I asked why they did not go directly to Group Hospital, which is ten minutes from their house. Mrs Polski explained:

> We went to see the doctor Monday, and he said: "Why didn't you take him to the hospital right away?" But in the book, they keep telling you: "Don't go to the hospital. Call up the Medical Center first, and the doctor will come and see you. If you need hospitalization they'll send you there." That's why we never bothered calling on Sunday, and that's why we waited. Otherwise I would have gone to the hospital. It's convenient from here. I could take him there in the car, which we did on Monday . . . then I know our doctor is in. Eleven o'clock is his first appointment.

On Monday morning the couple went to the doctor's office. After an electrocardiogram and examination the doctor instructed the Polskis to go right to the hospital. They did not. Once more over his wife's objections, the man drove home, put his car in the garage – because his wife "has trouble in the driveway." Only then did he call a friend to take him to the hospital.

Three elements can be identified in the above example as influencing care-seeking behavior. The first is the attempt to normalize the symptoms by treating them as a variation of a relatively minor, time-limited ailment. The persistance of this effort is remarkable against the evidence of a serious problem, a phenomenon which makes the study of denial such an important and fascinating one. The second element in the process involved – the interaction between the spouses. While Mrs Polski made suggestions and offered strong opinions as to what ought to be done in the situation, it was Mr Polski who controlled the timing of all events, from when to initiate help-seeking to when precisely to enter the medical system as a coronary patient. The third component involves the patient's knowledge of the routines and regulations of the medical care system they were members of, and the attitudes toward encountering that system.

The beginning of the crisis, then, involves people in a series of encounters: with self, significant others, and a medical bureaucracy. The experiences of another couple, Mr and Mrs Ambrosio, shed additional light on these encounters. Mr Ambrosio also described his symptoms as very painful, keeping him from sleep the entire night. Only the next morning, after exhausting the supply of over-the-counter medications they kept at home, did he ask his wife to call their physician. The call was actually made two hours after the realization of a need to get professional help. They waited until the physician's office hours began:

I thought, we thought, the center opened at ten. You couldn't, I guess, get emergency. Well, we were just waiting for ten for the center to open.

They were told to come to the center, where the doctor examined Mr Ambrosio and sent him to another part of the building for an electrocardiogram. They reported a half hour wait before a machine was available. When the family physician read the results of the electrocardiogram, he told the couple, "Possible coronary, go straight to the hospital." Mr Ambrosio asked the doctor if he could go home first. The doctor, I was told, adamantly refused. Nevertheless, outside the doctor's office Mr Ambrosio told his wife to take him home. She recalled this incident:

> So I am walking out with my husband to go to the car, which is parked in the lot there, at least 150 or 200 feet away. As we are walking, he says to me "I want you to take me home. I didn't shave" . . . and [he said he had to do] some other things. So I said, "I'm taking you to the hospital." He said: "I want to go home."

She won the argument and drove to the hospital. However, Mrs Ambrosio was not able to control the situation entirely. The doctor had explicitly stated that Mr Ambrosio was not to walk from the car to the emergency room once they arrived at the hospital, but should use a wheelchair. The following is what happened, as she recalled, when they arrived at Group Hospital:

> I knew where to stop, but there was a truck in front of me, and there were cars. They were tooting and tooting and there was no place to park. My husband opens the door and says, "Park the car." I say: "No, you are not going to walk, I'm getting the wheelchair." "Park the car!" he shouted.

He walked to the hospital while she parked the car.

Even after reaching the hospital and being admitted into the coronary care unit, the consequences of these events may remain a burden, particularly for the spouse who second guesses decisions made in the storm of crisis: A wife recalled:

> When we got into the ambulance, when he finally decided to let me call the ambulance, going to the hospital all I could think of is: "If I had only not listened to him. If I had called at 8:30. If I hadn't listened to him. Why did I listen to him? Look how many hours he's suffered. God knows what's going to be with now!" That's all I kept asking myself as the ambulance kept going. . . . As he was sitting here in this chair I should have gone to that telephone and not listened to him. So he would have fought me. He would have said I don't want you to. Still I should not have listened.

Unless the experiences of these people are unique and

ınrepresentative of the general experience of people in
hospital phase of their careers as heart patients and
of heart patients, the pathway to medical care is
...gely difficult to navigate. Patient and family must
traverse an unusual and difficult terrain with little guidance or
forewarning of the obstacles that they will meet on the way to
the coronary care unit. The journey to find the help that is so
urgently needed is undertaken under conditions of severe
physical, social, and psychological disability. The family
must mobilize for action when it is in a highly weakened state.
Notwithstanding the fact that individuals can and do rise to
the occasion, the group's normal channels of decision making
and mechanisms for problem solving are themselves
problematic.

It is interesting to note, in the examples given above, how
the men struggled to retain some control over how the
situation was being defined and acted out. In their efforts not
to withdraw from normal role behavior, they illustrate the
social context from which sick role behavior emerges.

The circuitous route to the hospital, which we have seen
can be detoured and delayed in various ways, reflects more
than just fear and denial (Hackett and Cassem 1969). The two
systems – family and medical – seem to lack knowledge of
each other, a situation Litwak and Meyer (1966) suggest is a
result of their incongruent structural properties. Interviews
with patients, spouses, and children reveal that when they
were ready to act they were uncertain about the routine to
follow in an unusual situation: whom to contact, when is it
appropriate to ask for help, how urgent is it to follow
instructions precisely. The families seemed not to be understood either. It seemed to be assumed that the lay definition of
the situation mirrored that of the professional. When the
physician directed Mr O'Shea, another of our subjects, to go
to the hospital for immediate care, he probably did not
anticipate that Mr Shea would first travel around to get his
wife and then his daughter to be with during the trip, which
again, was marred by conflict over who should do the driving.
This behavior reflects the psychosocial need for family
support, which can weigh as heavily as felt need for medical
care.

The Beginning of Research: Patients and Families

Patients and families, then, had to be recruited for the research on which this report is based at a time when the crisis was in an acute phase, physically and emotionally. Yet, as a practical matter, recruiting families into the study was surprisingly, yet deceptively, simple. I approached patients when, in the judgment of the nurse-in-charge of the ICU, they could tolerate being interviewed. Because I was a participant observer on the intensive care unit, I was myself observed by patients and visitors as I attended medical rounds, interviewed patients and staff, and took notes of what transpired during the course of the day and evening. Prospective patients therefore had the opportunity to learn of the research process even before they were formally requested to take part. So when it came time for me to enlist prospective patients, some had already formed an impression of me and my work. Only one patient refused to take part in the research. Recruiting other family members was only slightly more complicated, and only two would not agree to enter into a study in which their actions and feelings would be made known to a relative stranger for a period of several months.

Interviewing patients in the Intensive Care Unit presented a few logistical problems. The patients themselves seemed ready, even eager, to talk. Staff members were uniformly cooperative. Privacy for interviewing was lacking, however, since most beds were only several feet apart. While drawing the curtain around the patient's bed provided a visual barrier, anyone who was interested in listening in could have overheard the interview. Open ended interviewing gave the patients some control and the option of protecting their privacy. The interviewer tried to be sensitive to questions that might embarrass the subject. In spite of the limitations of the setting for interviewing, a good deal of information was able to be gained by this method. Some men seemed to derive considerable benefit from unburdening themselves of worries; others seemed cheered to describe the situation they were in, particularly the incongurities they found in it, or the things they found unusual and amusing. I learned that one need not tread too gently; the patients had little difficulty discussing their illnesses, their fears, and their concerns. Other research with coronary patients (Cowie 1976) suggests that one of the needs such patients have is to understand the factors that contributed to the illness and to construct a sequence of events and circumstances that "make sense." Possibly, the interviews helped the men to work through this process.

Family members were initially quite eager to establish contact with the researcher. They showed much interest in the project, and some even observed that they and the patients would benefit from talking about their experiences. However, not all were as eager to go beyond the initial contact and actually begin the interviews. One gets the impression that in this situation the researcher fulfills a need people have to be taken account of by a medical system that often is too busy caring for the illness to notice the emotional needs of the victim and his grief-stricken loved ones. Being asked to participate in a research project may be interpreted on some level as meaning: I have been noticed, singled out, have not been forgotten. Saying yes to the researcher may only affirm a need for recognition, for connectedness within the acute care setting. Perhaps because of my proximity to the patient, my access to staff, my sheer presence in and about the unit, I was perceived by families as someone who could provide them with the contact they desired. On one particular occasion, as I was leaving the Intensive Care Unit, I heard someone call after me: "Are you a doctor?" I turned and noticed the wife of a patient who had been admitted to the ICU that morning. She was sitting on a folding chair just beyond the ICU door, looking quite distraught. I answered her that I was not a physician and continued down the hall. She called after me: "You look like a doctor." I went to her and introduced myself. She told me of her husband and expressed her fears about his chances of survival. I listened and tried to comfort her. Yet when I suggested we sit down and talk more about it, perhaps over some coffee, she declined, saying she just wanted to go home.

Although family members expressed no reservations about being interviewed at home, when it was explained prior to their consenting, it only occurred in half the cases. The others preferred that we talk in the hospital when they came to visit. It was not easy arranging these interviews, however. With some it was necessary to reiterate the rationale for interviews while the patients were in the hospital. Before long it became clear that initial willingness to participate in the research did not mean that family members either understood completely what was being asked of them or were able to make any specific commitments at a time of such anxiety and uncertainty. Reflecting on the situation, it is understandable that people whose attention is riveted on the present will have difficulty conceptualizing a research project that intends to look at the process of adjustment. In the acute phase of crisis, it may be hard to relate to someone who is interested in the long haul. In discussing the research with families, I tended to emphasize later stages of the career and may have given the impression of not being interested in their immediate concerns. At the time, I felt this was the more sensitive approach, although I have since come to think that my own conflicts about illness and dying may have influenced my judgment. As I was to learn, these people were not so much in need of being protected against their feelings as they were of having someone to talk with, when ready to do so, about the reality of their current situation.

Remember too, that the sudden event of illness had profoundly upset the flow of their lives. Although life revolved around ICU visiting hours, the basic tasks of daily living had to be attended. It was difficult for people to establish a schedule. So much was happening; there were so many things to think about. There was no indication that anyone regretted consenting to the study. I saw these people regularly in and outside of the ICU, and we always spoke for a while. But it was indicated by half that home visits would be difficult and that, while they would be willing to talk, they could not be precise about when they could do this. Under these circumstances, the researcher must not add to the family's burdens. Yet he is obliged to seek the knowledge his study requires. In the present instance, two strategies were employed. One simply involved waiting, putting in long hours at the hospital in order to be available when the wives and children were ready to talk at length. I did not press individuals to meet with me beyond telling them that I was eager to do so when they were ready. The other was a more active approach. Many of the wives at times used public transportation in reaching the hospital. All were grateful for the offer of a ride home by the researcher, who used the opportunity to interview them. Finlayson and McEwen (1977:61) seem to have encountered a similar problem with some of the spouses of heart patients in their study and utilized a similar solution. They arranged for those who worked full time and were on tight schedules to be driven to the hospital before visiting hours in order to make time for the interview.

Being solicitous of subjects' needs serves more of a purpose than securing interview time. Certainly, concern on the part of any researcher puts his subjects at ease and allays fears that can be expected to arise as to whether the research will be a burden to the patient or family members. But for a naturalistic study such as this one, it also sets a tone: this will be a cooperative venture between subject and researcher, and both will play active roles. For the researcher wanting to study lives in progress, he or she must shape his design to fit the contours of the experience as it actually exists. In my case, I was seeking a privileged position with the families by being allowed access to members in the hospital and home in order to observe them and talk with them about how they were handling matters some of which were mundane, others highly intimate. I had a few preconceived notions of where precisely to look and what to ask, which would give me the understanding that I sought. I was depending on *them* to tell *me*! For the families, scheduling time for interviews, interacting with a social scientist-researcher made additional demands on time and energy and was, in fact, one more circumstance brought about by the heart attack which had to be managed. To have attempted to impose a schedule on these people, or to have been emotionally neutral in dealing with them, would have established the subject–researcher relationship on an inappropriate basis.

Skillful fieldworkers such as William Whyte (1943), Elliot Liebow (1967), and Rosalie Wax (1971) acknowledge the debt their work owes to subjects such as Doc, who, as Whyte

(1943:301) reported, "became, in a very real sense, a collaborator in the research." All subjects need not be, cannot be, on such close terms with the investigator. Yet, the best data will be produced when subjects permit the researcher to enter their world. The assumption that guided my approach was that the extent to which this occurred would depend on three factors: subjects' understanding of the purposes of the research, their perception of the researcher's concern for the patient and the needs of the family, and the researcher's flexibility.

This raises the question of how much the researcher ought to become involved with his subjects. Will he record events dispassionately, deliberately avoiding any direct response to these same events in order not to influence them by his presence. Or will he, like a friend, be helpful without being intrusive and show concern for their affairs. I believe one can accomplish the latter without either compromising the objectivity of one's perspective or intruding upon the prerogatives of others, including the primary physician. Liebow (1967:253), discussing his relationship with the streetcorner men he studied, made an important point in this regard: "I usually tried to limit money or other favors to what I thought each would have gotten from another friend had he the same resources as I. I tried to meet requests as best I could without becoming conspicuous." I too was prepared to help out where I could. Although I did not formulate strict guidelines prior to meeting the families, some did emerge out of the situations I was faced with. I offered help when my actions could not change anyone's plans, only make it easier to carry them out – driving someone to the doctor's office, for example. I responded to their uncertainty by providing information. For example, when a spouse reported being perplexed over the diet her husband was following in the hospital and would have to follow at home, I informed her that the hospital had a dietitian on staff whose job it was to explain such things. When people either directly or indirectly asked my advice, I tried to respond as intelligently as I could, and when this meant responding to questions about the patient's medical condition or any aspects of his treatment, I did so by suggesting that the person ask the nurse or doctor at the next visit. I did not intervene with members of medical or nursing staffs on behalf of any of the members of my study. In other words, I did not ask their questions for them or refer a nurse to anyone, even if I thought such a meeting ought to take place. I did not view my role as that of a counselor or member of the therapeutic team. I did, however, try to act as a friend who in time of need tries to comfort by offering practical help and advice when there is an obvious need, and who listens sympathetically and non-judgmentally to someone's concerns. I did not criticize men who resumed smoking against their physician's orders, even when this occurred in the hospital. If, however, I learned that someone was, through ignorance, placing himself in immediate danger, I would have intervened.

Beginning of Research: Medical and Nursing Staff

I did not begin approaching patients or family members about entering the study until I had experienced the hospital, especially the ICU, for a couple of months as an observer. This was probably fortunate for my subjects because I had much more of a grasp of their problems, particularly those having to do with managing the medical care system, by the time I did meet them and could be more sensitive in dealing with them. This study got under way by interviewing doctors and nurses and by observing around the hospital, with the focus being the sites where the two institutions, family and hospital, met: the emergency room and the Intensive Care Unit. It was in the Intensive Care Unit that one could observe meaningful interaction within the healing triad of staff-patient-family..

In this nine-bed ICU, nurses reigned. There were, in fact, no physicians who were permanently assigned to the unit. Physicians were actually on the unit either for scheduled medical/nursing rounds or when called by nurses to look into the condition of a particular patient. In contrast, nurses were present continually and assisted physicians when the latter did hands-on care. Physicians came onto the unit for specific purposes and left when their business was finished. For the nurses the ICU was their domain. To a significant degree it was the nursing staff that set the tone, professionally by initiating house staff visits there, and socially by controlling many of the important conditions under which informal social interaction took place. The only non-patient space, the nursing station and the lounge, clearly "belonged to" the nurses, who used these spaces all day. Physicians had a right to be there to conduct their business, but if they socialized there they did so as the nurses' guests. When physicians observed me on the unit, at the nursing station, it was obvious to them that the legitimation for my presence had already been established.

Moreover, when I attended medical rounds, which were daily exercises led by the medical director and chief of cardiology, legitimation was confirmed. My presence on the ICU did not, therefore, provoke any objections from physicians, at least none that I was aware of. Actually, most physicians whom I spoke with in the hospital, and who observed me as I them, expressed interest in the study and found the time to be interviewed when asked. I was never asked to restrict my observations or my note taking for that matter. Armed with lab coat and clip board, I observed at will patient examinations and interactions among medical and nursing staffs and patients. Significantly, I was able to learn in a direct fashion the medical plans for patients, including instructions given them regarding their activities of daily living while on the unit. This proved to be invaluable for providing a frame of reference for observations of these same patients later in the day. As with members of the patients' families, it helped to know the physicians' schedules – when they took breaks, went to dinner, and when things were slow. What added to my legitimacy was the fact that I was already a part of the ICU scene when new house staff arrived. Compared with them, I was an insider.

To at least a few members of the house staff, my familiarity with the unit and the knowledge I had acquired of the literature on the psychosocial dimensions of coronary heart disease etiology and rehabilitation made me someone they could talk to about some of the issues they dealt with in their work. For the most part, these referred to matters of a general nature, which staff in all ICUs have to deal with, such as patient denial or patient adjustment to the ICU environment, and could be discussed in terms of what the literature says or whether or not some abstract concept applies.

Occasionally, however, I was sought out to play a consultation role in the management of a real problem with a real patient. One such situation involved a patient with a very poor prognosis and who, in the resident's mind, showed signs of cognitive impairment. The resident asked me to listen as he tried to explain to the patient the surgical option that was available to him and then to help to assess the patient's capacity to understand what was being said. My response was that this kind of direct involvement in the physician–patient relationship would be inappropriate, going far beyond the bounds of my role in this ICU. The experience taught me to be wary lest the distinction between participant and participant observer became blurred.

When I sat at the nursing station there was little that I could not see on the unit. The station itself was a long narrow table, half of which held monitors so that nurses could keep the patients' heart rhythms under close scrutiny by either looking at the station or at the same apparatus at the bedside. The other half was workspace for the staff. It was rarely unoccupied. The station commanded a view not only of every patient on the unit but also of the door of the unit and the waiting area beyond. From the outset I had, in a rudimentary way, the same view of the unit as the staff had, which, I believe, encouraged the nurses to take an interest in what I was observing and recording. They responded with alacrity to my requests to understand what the unit did. It was made clear that I was free to see things up close, including procedures such as pacemaker insertions and emergency resuscitation of patients in cardiac arrest. ICU nurses were remarkably open in explaining their work with patients and exhibited a high degree of self confidence in their nursing abilities. However, my attention to what they thought to be mundane and trivial, like whether the unit was quiet or noisy, or how often in the course of an hour patients and nurses spoke to each other, provoked occasional queries as to what I was "really" looking for. Even after I had been on the unit for some time, I could see that some were bothered when I attempted to step back and describe the ambience at a particular point in time. Beyond the fact that almost anyone would react to being watched in this way, one needs to realize that under normal conditions the ICU nurses were highly visible. There was almost no place one could go without being in view of the nursing station. Likewise, voices easily carried across the room. Nurses stayed on the unit for the duration of their shift, with only a lunch break to provide a change of environment. It is no wonder, given the already high observability of staff members, that some found the additional scrutiny particularly burdensome (see also Coser 1961). I could think of no way of handling this except to be as open as possible about the aims of my work and being discreet in taking notes. I tried not to hide the fact that I was recording what I saw and talked about with staff, even if I did not do so at the time. I often used the small staff lounge which was adjacent to the medication cabinet for my writing. I also attempted in various ways to enter into the life of the unit. When I had the opportunity to lend a hand with something, I did not hesitate. I took an interest in staff members' career plans and shared stories of family and social life.

Having described the reactions of others to my presence, I must also say something of my own problems in adapting to the hospital setting. For the neophyte, the ICU can be a jarring experience. There is a very definite sensory barrier which one confronts immediately upon entering the unit. The sights, sounds, and smells one encounters give the unmistakeable impression of sickness. The odor of medication and body waste pervades the area. Sounds of labored breathing, of oxygen and ventilators, the deep sighs and moans which come from each corner of what seems to be a very small room for so much sickness, the hum of machinery, blend together in one continuous lament. Coming into the unit one goes from daylight to dusk; lights are kept dimmed; the natural light of day does not enter the unit to give one a sense of times. All around are the tools of treatment. Posted like sentries, the defibrillating machines stand ready for emergency duty. Above each patient is a screen upon which a bead of light traces a pattern by which trained staff monitor the functioning of the heart. At the nursing station the doctors and nurses examine data tapes from the patients' monitors. My initial reaction was to feel uncertain about basic forms of social intercourse, for I felt I was in a place where the familiar, taken-for-granted assumptions that give one bearings in the "normal" world did not apply. I felt confused and angered by the laughter and small talk coming from the nursing station. I thought: how could anyone be worldly in this subculture of stricken people? I wanted to see expressed in the actions of doctors and nurses what I felt when I experienced the environment. I know I refrained from joining in some of the socializing in the unit because I felt it was inappropriate. I failed at the outset to appreciate the value of this behavior as a coping mechanism for the staff and as a relief for the patients.

I found my own standards of modesty, privacy, and propriety clashed with some of what I saw on the unit. While this made me uncomfortable, I feel it sharpened my awareness of what other outsiders, such as spouses, children, friends, and relatives of patients must feel as well.

Fortunately, there were structured activities like medical/nursing rounds that provided guidance for my orientation to the unit. The nursing station also provided me with a vantage point and a secure base from which to learn how patients would react to me and my questions about how they felt to be in this place, and how I would react to them up close.

What This Book is About

Process

We shall explore eight examples of how heart attack affects inter-personal relationships and personal identity. The events which will be described took place within a three- to four-month period. Other studies of long-term effects of heart attack have followed patients for a year and even longer and have concluded that in some cases adjustment occurs for an indeterminate period. The present study, therefore, cannot claim to be comprehensive, either in terms of the time period covered or the topics that are addressed, since changes brought about by an illness that is both life threatening and chronic are likely to have a host of psychological and sociological consequences for the victim and his significant others.

In the period that was observed, however, the families faced both the immediate threat of death and the necessity to emerge from crisis and begin the process of resuming activities that are essential for normal social and psychological functioning. While relatively brief when measured in time, this period is rich in experiences that are critical to long-term adjustment. In a few months, the families lived through several identifiable stages of crisis and adjustment, two of which have been cited: the pretreatment phase of problem definition, and the formal entry into the medical care system.

For the duration of the stay in the Intensive Care Unit, which can last from several days to several weeks, the patient has little contact with anyone except the medical staff and other patients. Direct interaction with family members is limited to very brief periods – measured in minutes – a few times daily. While the patient is in the ICU, the family must live with the possibility of death, since the prevention of events that can easily threaten the life of the weakened heart-attack victim is the explicit mission of the ICU. Separately, patient and family must each catch hold of the fast-moving events and begin to interpret them, to define the situation.

As the site of care moves to another less controlled setting in the hospital, so must the concern of patient and family shift. Two social processes are central in the post-ICU phase of hospitalization. First of all, patient and family are rejoined after a period that has been and continues to be stressful, which has presented each with distinct images and impressions. In order to communicate effectively each must learn the other's definition of the situation, particularly in relation to each other's expectations for present and future behavior. Second, since the patient will not return home cured, but at home will be expected to comply with a prescribed regimen, the details of the condition and nuances of the treatment can no longer be the domain of the medical staff alone. Moreover, since the family will be expected to play an important role in carrying forth the treatment regimen, the members must

decide prior to hospital discharge what must be done and how
to arrange the family routine in order to accomplish what
needs to be done. The requirement of the situation is that the
family unit be active and future-oriented in contrast to the
passive and present-oriented nature of the previous situation.
Once home, the focus returns to the present as the family
copes with the immediate problems of operationalizing the
regimen as each member of the group has understood and
interpreted it. Together, patient and family struggle in
uncertainty and fear to make the recovery work. In the
absence of ever present medical expertise, decisions about the
details of care loom large. Death fear may return.

There is another challenge presented in the immediate
post-hospital period, namely role adjustment. The shift of
the locus of care into the home does not bring with it a
substantial change in the sick role of the person who has
suffered the heart attack; he remains a patient. The obligations of the well family members do change, however. They
replace the hospital personnel and may be seen as incurring
nurse–surrogate roles. The dynamics of family interaction
during this period center around the solution of the husband-
patient, wife/child-nurse conflict. A theoretical basis for this
conflict has been offered by Parsons and Fox (1952), and a
summary of their thesis is presented later in this chapter. We
will suggest that differences between families in the way this
conflict is worked out can be explained to a significant extent
by factors related to family social structure and value
orientation. As time works its healing effects and strength
returns to men's bodies, the family must come to grips with
the individual and collective changes the illness has necess-
itated. Heart disease is the premier example of the effect of
lifestyle on physical health (Enelow and Henderson 1974).
Recovery from, and prevention of, subsequent coronary
illness requires changes in various areas of behavior having
to do with diet, exercise, and emotional stress. For some these
changes raise questions about areas of life that are of
significant social and psychological importance, such as work.
The person who is recovering is not the only one who has a
stake in the process of returning to normal social functioning.
In all intimate groups, a change in the status of one member

affects the others. Everyone has a stake in the outcome of the recovery process, and each person brings his individual perspective to the collective struggle to determine what will return to a pre-illness state.

The question of how people can best recover from heart attack and return to a full and active life has received a considerable amount of attention from medical and social scientists. Empirical data collected in the course of numerous scientific studies of the physiological, psychological, and sociological determinants of recovery have changed the way we think about treating and rehabilitating heart attack victims. No longer are patients confined to bed rest for long periods of time. Early mobilization after the initial attack, once avoided, is now encouraged by modern medical norms (Tucker *et al.* 1973). The patient's *perception* of his health has been recognized as a key variable, along with objective health status, influencing successful reentry into the world of work (Garrity 1973). Research has also found that the social and emotional support received at home from those who care for his needs and who share the burden of the illness and recovery makes a significant contribution to the patient's wellbeing (Croog, Levine, Lurie 1968). The structure of the family itself and its characteristic ways of coping with difficulties make a real difference in the outcome of the recovery process (Hansen and Hill 1964: 811–15).

In spite of the attention that has been paid to the broad issues of physical and psychosocial recovery from this and other illnesses, Bermann (1973:64) is correct in saying that "the territory of family stress is almost uncharted with respect to interactional processes in the face of disruptive forces . . ." By documenting the first-hand experiences of family members who have lived through the disruptive aftermath of serious illness, the present study identifies significant interactional processes not only within families but between families and the health care system which characterize the efforts of families to attain a full measure of physical and psychosocial recovery. This study may assist those who design treatment modalities to gain an awareness of the problems people face at different stages of a crisis and to appreciate how a health care system can accentuate the strengths and weaknesses of the average family faced with serious illness.

The present work will amplify existing knowledge of the processes involved in recovering from heart disease. It is particularly relevant to studies of recovery that take a longitudinal perspective, such as the recent work of Croog and Levine (1977) and Finlayson and McEwen (1977). These studies, which utilized larger samples, successfully documented the changes that occur in peoples' lives following a heart attack and have identified processes of family dynamics and personality structure that predispose certain outcomes. Yet these quantitative studies leave us to wonder about the day-to-day lives in the homes of the people they studied, about the human emotions that are measured, but not described, by their statistics. While studies have taken the measure of family functioning at different points in time, we shall explore the time in between in order to learn how relationships which are damaged by a heart attack are renewed.

Two concepts are central to this type of analysis. One is "career", which, as Goffman (1961:127) explains, refers "to any social strand of any person's course through life . . . changes over time as are basic and common to the members of a social category . . ." It is to chart the course taken through a significant segment of the career of the heart attack victim and his immediate family that is the task of this work. We shall do so by considering not just the idiosyncratic responses to the crisis (which are important in their own right!), but those that reflect the way that medical care for heart attack is socially organized.

The second concept is W.I. Thomas's (1928) notion of "definition of the situation." As I have tried to indicate, the onset of heart attack unleashes forces that create fear and terrible uncertainty for both the victim and his family. Finlayson and McEwen (1977:169) describe the initial period as like a vacuum where usual ways of thinking and acting cannot be applied. How do people in such a situation develop the understanding required to cope with the immediate emotional impact and the changes in their lives that will result? What images and symbols are employed, what information is conveyed, what transactions occur to give bearing to these people in crisis?

Relationships

Throughout this work we shall be exploring interpersonal relationship at various levels. Certainly, relations among members of the eight nuclear families will provide a critical focus of the analysis. However, we shall also be concerned with relationships between family members – patients, spouses, children – and members of the health care team, particularly nurses and doctors.

When dealing with family members, a great deal of attention was paid to events that in some way were connected to the illness itself or to some circumstance created by the illness. Things in the lives of people that did not seem significantly affected by the illness were given much less attention. An example of something relatively unexplored in this analysis is the nuclear family's relations with its kinship network, except when kin had a significant effect on transactions among members of the family around some illness-related issue.

Something else the reader should note is that we will be exploring events among members of the same household. Little primary data came from children, married or single, who lived apart from their parents. This then will be a detailed look at a portion of family life during a delimited period of crisis and significant change occurring to those most affected on a day-to-day basis.

Studies of family life during episodes of illness indicate that the most pervasive change the group has to deal with involves role behavior (Anthony 1970; Bell 1966; Jacobson and Eichhorn 1964; Strauss 1975). The withdrawal through illness of one family member from normal role behavior necessitates a shift on the part of other role players in the family to accomodate the loss of function. While families can and do manage this change without experiencing severe disruption of functioning, shifts in what people can do and be responsible for may under certain circumstances be accompanied by interpersonal conflict as new arrangements are negotiated by members. Feelings of personal loss of competency and self-esteem may surface on account of a perceived diminution of social worth. Rosenstock and Kutner (1969:652) have pointed out that role shifts following crisis

within the family can have an alienating effect when one
member no longer perceives that his own social and psychological needs can be met under the prevailing arrangements of
responsibility and authority in the family. One form which
such alienation may take, these authors suggest, is "retreat-
ism," defined as "the voluntary or involuntary separation of
alienated members from one another or from the rest of the
family, or the social and psychological withdrawal of the
members even though they are physically present."

Some family units come through a period of crisis in better
shape than existed previously. Hansen and Hill (1964:790)
have argued that this may occur more frequently than is
apparent from empirical studies because of a tendency on the
part of researchers to emphasize, even reify, "system"
concepts, such as equilibrium and homeostasis. This tends to
obscure occasions of "system enhancement." What Hansen
and Hill suggest is that people have the capacity to use crises
and turn them into opportunities "which *release* them,
individually and in their intimate relationships, to develop
arrangements that are ordered more closely to their particular
needs."

It may also be the case that the changes introduced by a
crisis such as serious illness may be beneficial for some, but
not all, members of a group. Even as the collectivity, the
family as an entity, struggles to create a new balance, certain
individuals may experience enhanced opportunities for self-
fulfillment. Furthermore, and this may be difficult for even
longitudinal surveys to pick up, a family may have a series of
experiences, some of which are characterized by conflict and
disorganization and some by a heightened sense of mutuality
and cohesion. Hill (1958) likens the course of adjustment to
crisis to the path of a roller coaster. This is all to suggest that
the "typical" reaction of a family under stress may well
involve both positive and negative outcomes over time with
various impacts for different members. As we follow events in
our eight families, we shall see some of these patterns emerge.

Social Structure

The question of how characteristic patterns of interaction

within the family are related to qualities of coping with crisis is important for both theoretical and pragmatic reasons. Are some forms of living together more adaptive to change and resilient under stress than others? Can rehabilitation strategies be tailored to the coping styles that predominate in certain identifiable types of families? There is some evidence that the answer to these questions is in the affirmative. In summarizing her data from a study of how family structure affects health behavior, Pratt (1976:137-38) states: "it is the family's overall pattern of arrangements for relating to, and working with, each other which is important. Specifically, the pattern that tends to contribute to health is one in which members are given freedom and are encouraged in their efforts to cope and to function." Finlayson and McEwen (1977:173) have reported that poor outcomes tended to be associated with "traditional" style marriages rather than "partnership" marriages and with men who had "previously been intensively committed to instrumental roles and lacking ability in expressive ones." Litman (1966) in a case-control study comparing persons who adjusted well to a physical rehabilitation program to those who had a poor response, found that those in the former category were likely to live in highly integrated families which supported their rehabilitative efforts.

In the present study we attempt to demonstrate how different styles of inter-personal behavior and patterns of role playing typical of normal living may give rise to certain ways of handling problems in living together in the aftermath of an illness crisis. We cannot predict from this study the prevalence of any particular mode of adaptation in the population, but rather suggest that where certain patterns of instrumental and affective relations are present, characteristic patterns of adjustment behavior may follow.

Interaction across Systems

Analyses of careers must deal with the interaction of the person with the institutions that structure the career pathway. Since we are dealing with processes of adjustment and coping of family units, we have attempted to uncover the nature of interaction between the family and the medical care bureaucracy. Again, there are both theoretical and pragmatic reasons for this.

Over the years, the major institutions of society have become increasingly specialized. As Rodman (1969:96) explains, "not only has economic production been taken over by other organizations than the family . . . the schools, the mass media, peer groups, hospitals, voluntary associations, etc., have taken over functions formerly performed by the family." In the modern era, the family acts as a kind of emotional shock absorber. Goode (1963:14) explains this:

> The modern technological system is psychologically burdensome on the individual because it demands an unremitting discipline. To the extent that evaluation is based on achievement and universalism, the individual gets little emotional security from his work. . . . The conjugal family again integrates with such a system by its emphasis on emotionality, especially in the relationship of husband and wife. It has the task of restoring the imput-output emotional balance of individualism in such a job structure.

In this context Parsons and Fox (1952) have presented the classical functionalist interpretation for the separation of the health care function from the home. They point out that the relationship between a patient and the persons caring for him departs from the normal pattern among adults in family life. In its dependence and in its freedom from normal responsibilities, the patient role is a privileged one, and has some attributes of the child role. In a society as demanding as ours, this privileged position might be sought as a welcome substitute for normally stressful role obligations. Ideally, the role of healer in society deals with this contingency. First, by encouraging the patient to suspend his attachment to adult concerns, he elicits the patient's trust. Then, as the treatment takes effect, he withdraws support for dependency and offers approval for a return to normal role responsibilities. Were family members to share in the therapeutic process, their emotional connections to the patient would, in the Parsons-Fox analysis, make it difficult to maintain the required objectivity and affective neutrality. More often, the tendency on the part of the family members would be to overindulge the patient, thus inviting him to perpetuate his illness; or, to be overly strict, and intolerant of the patient's dependency. In either case, the tensions introduced by the illness would be compounded.

With the increasing chronicity of illness in our society and the emphasis on early hospital discharge and home-based care for a variety of conditions, it is clear that we must develop strategies for making homes more suitable places to provide health care. Families can no longer be thought of as being outside of the therapeutic process. Bringing families back in, however, may not be an uncomplicated task, especially given the increased bureaucratization of modern health care. It has been argued that not only are there sharp differences in the basic social structure of primary groups and bureaucracies, they have "antithetical mutually destructive atmospheres" (Litwak and Meyer, 1966:35).

This raises important questions for our analysis of family response to the illness crisis, especially after the patient returns from the hospital to complete his recovery at home. If primary groups (here, the family) and bureaucratic organiz- ations (here, a complex medical care system) have "mutually destructive atmospheres," is it possible to expect the family adequately to operationalize the expectations and prescrip- tions of the medical care system with regard to the patient's regimen of care and treatment at home? What problems are in store for current medical care innovations such as programs that aim to reduce the time patients spend in the hospital and that would place greater emphasis on home-based treatment thereby expanding the role of the family in the treatment process? Can family members be expected to take on func- tions once exclusively performed in a hospital by pro- fessionals? Can a family work with a health care bureaucracy in a systematic, mutually supportive effort to restore a person's health?

Even in the acute phase of illness when patients are hospitalized, the importance of the family's relationship with the caregiving system cannot be overlooked. As Davis (1963:57) learned from his long-term study of polio victims, "the hospital and its treatment procedures are the agents that

reshape and redefine the recovery orientation of the family."
In other words, hospitalization is an experience that shapes
attitudes toward self in relation to the illness, a consequence
reaching beyond the immediate physical ailment into the
depth of the individual psyche and collective consciousness.

The Families

In Chapter 4 the structure of each family's interior life will be
addressed. However, since in the next two chapters, dealing
with the experience of hospitalization, the reader will find
material taken directly from patients and family members, I
have prepared a profile of each family which contains enough
background information to insure that the people mentioned
will not appear as strangers to the reader.

The eight families are similar in some respects. All the
members are white. No one at the time gave evidence of
significant emotional disturbance. Nor was there any indication of alcoholism, drug addiction, or other condition that
would place someone outside of what is commonly considered to be normal limits. The families lived in residential
neighborhoods of one of the nation's major cities.

The Ambrosios

Mr and Mrs Ambrosio are in their mid sixties and both are
retired. He had a middle management position with the
municipal Bureau of Standards. He does some consulting
with local business on compliance with municipal regulations. She is a former legal secretary who continues to do
occasional *per diem* work. The couple have two married
children and live alone in their own home.

Mr Ambrosio has no prior history of heart disease. He is
diabetic and takes medication for the condition. He had not
been following the diet regimen prescribed by his physician.
In the past year he seems to have had more minor ailments
such as colds, flu symptoms, and the like than previously.
Mrs Ambrosio has a chronic condition called osteoarthritis
which is a degenerative joint disease which, in her case, affects
the lower back and occasionally causes her to limit her

activities. Both spouses have received medical care from the same physician for more than ten years.

Both lead active lives. They have hobbies and other interests which keep them busy in and out of the home. They regularly socialize with friends in the neighborhood, are active in community affairs, and maintain contact with their married children.

The Astis

Mr and Mrs Asti are in their late fifties. He is a foreman for a construction company. She is not employed outside of the home but is seriously considering looking for a clerical position. Two of the three Asti children are unmarried and live at home. Rose is nineteen years old and attends a local college; John is twenty and is a construction worker. The married daughter lives with her husband and children in an apartment in the family home.

Mr Asti has no prior history of heart disease. He does have a history of hypertension but has not maintained the medication regimen and has had no recent physician contact. Mrs Asti reported no active health problems. In the months prior to the heart attack both spouses felt well and were following a normal routine except for the fact that they were planning a vacation trip to another state, a novel experience for the couple. The family maintains active contact with a number of relatives who live nearby. The children have active social lives with their own friends.

The Goldbergs

Mr and Mrs Goldberg are in their early sixties. He is retired from a job with a roofing contractor, although he takes occasional jobs on his own. She has not worked outside the home. Both spouses have married children from previous marriages. They live by themselves in their own home in which they rent an apartment to tenants.

Mr Goldberg has no prior history of heart disease, although several days prior to his heart attack he felt poorly and saw his physician who took an electrocardiogram. At this time the couple was also planning to take a vacation trip.

The couple lives a quiet life centered around home and are not very much involved in community activities. They do maintain active contact with her son. Relations with his daughter have been strained for a while.

The Grassos

Mr and Mrs Grasso are in their mid fifties. He operates a family owned grocery store in the neighborhood, and she is a secretary for a large corporation. A twenty-four-year-old son, Anthony, was recently divorced and now lives at home. The couple has another married son.

Six years ago Mr Grasso suffered his first heart attack. He has not followed his physician's advice regarding diet or smoking. In fact, he has seen his physician only infrequently over the last year. He reported feeling well in the months preceeding the latest heart attack. Mrs Grasso has no active illnesses. Both spouses have used the same physician for more than ten years.

The couple have a very active social life with family and a large group of friends with whom they regularly socialize. Evenings and weekends tend to be very busy with Mr Grasso tending to business matters, Mrs Grasso catching up on housework, and both either entertaining or visiting friends and relatives. The couple own their own home and rent an apartment to tenants.

The O'Sheas

Mr and Mrs O'Shea are in their early sixties. He is a train conductor for the municipal transportation system. She works in the kitchen of a large restaurant. Of the couple's three children, one daughter who is soon to be married lives at home, one is married, and the other is single and lives out of state. The couple and their daughter are apartment dwellers.

Mr O'Shea has no prior history of heart disease, but about a week prior to the heart attack Mr O'Shea went to his regular physician complaining of chest discomfort. An electrocardiogram was scheduled for the next week. He was hospitalized before it occurred. Mrs O'Shea has hypertension, but otherwise reported being in general good health.

Mr O'Shea is very active in the affairs of his community, Mrs O'Shea much less so. Both, however, socialize with friends and maintain active contact with their married son.

The Polskis

Mr and Mrs Polski are in their early sixties. He is retired from the municipal transportation system where he worked as a mechanic. Mrs Polski has not been employed outside of the home. The couple have one married son and maintain two homes, one in the city and a smaller one in a distant suburb which they planned to give to their son as soon as Mr Polski finished putting an extention on it. He plans to build another home nearby the one the son will move into.

About ten years ago, Mr Polski was hospitalized for coronary insufficiency, a condition caused by inadequate coronary circulation which results in anginal pain. He reported no limitations as a result of this condition and in the year prior to the heart attack felt good. Mrs Polski's only health problem is a slight arthritic condition in her hands which occasionally causes her to curtail sewing and embroidering which are her hobbies.

Mr and Mrs Polski attend social functions at their church. However, Mr Polski's major activity is finishing the construction of his second home; Mrs Polski has a set of friends she sees regularly.

The Steins

Mr and Mrs Stein are in their late fifties. He is employed as a photoengraver, she as a secretary. The couple live by themselves in their own home, and have two married children.

Mr Stein has no prior history of heart disease and was not feeling unwell in the months preceeding the heart attack. Mrs Stein, however, has been under a doctor's care for a heart condition.

The couple's social life is somewhat limited by the fact that

Mr Stein works evenings and she works days. On weekends, the couple spend much of their time at home. They maintain active contact with their children and other relatives.

The Warrens

Mr and Mrs Warren are both in their mid sixties and retired. He worked as a automotive mechanic, she as a bank clerk. They have no children. Mr Warren drives a taxi one day a week.

Mr Warren has no prior history of heart disease. Except for a hiatus hernia which occasionally causes discomfort, Mr Warren felt good in the months preceeding the heart attack. Mrs Warren reported herself in good health with no active illnesses. The Warrens have had the same physician for close to ten years. When the heart attack struck, the couple were in the process of purchasing a retirement home in another state.

The couple lead a very quiet life with occasional socializing with friends and at church functions. They spend the bulk of their time in and around their home.

2

Social Structure and Social Behavior on an Intensive Care Unit*

Patient–Family Perspectives

There is a substantial body of literature focusing on the period following the onset of the heart attack in which the patient is cared for in an intensive care setting. Much of this writing addresses the phenomenon of delay in seeking professional help once symtoms appear (Hackett and Cassem 1969), as well as the problem of anxiety (Dominian and Dobson 1969; Cay *et al.* 1972) after the patient is diagnosed and sent to a coronary care unit. Studies examining the question of whether the critical care setting is stressful for patients often emphasize in their design the matter of transferring to another ward from the ICU (Minckley 1979). Numerous other articles have dealt with the problems encountered by staff members in coping with the strains inherent in this particular setting (Coombs and Goldman 1973; Vreeland and Ellis 1969; Michaels 1971; Obier and Haywood 1972). By and large, this literature has been about the emotional impact the situation has on the individuals involved. Less attention has been given to how patients *define* the situation and to how the social organization of the care setting influences the way in which people *perceive* and *interpret*, that is, give meaning to, the events in which they are suddenly caught up. Yet, it is these perceptions and definitions that will influence the strategies that are employed to cope with the problem. This takes cognizance of the fact that the heart patient in the ICU is at an early stage of what will be

* Pages 31–47 were first published in *Social Work and Health Care* 6 (2), and appear by kind permission of the publishers, The Haworth Press. All rights reserved.

an extended patient *career* (Goffman 1961) and that the ICU is an entry point into an extended system of care. The perspective that the patient gains on his condition at one point in his career is likely to affect how he approaches subsequent ones. Cowie (1976:87), who hypothesized that "the patient's subsequent adaptation to his heart attack would be influenced by events in his proto-patient career and his experiences in the hospital" has demonstrated the considerable extent to which hospitalized patients engaged in retrospective constructions of their own biographies in order to understand and make intelligible the crisis which had befallen them. Other authors have suggested that what the heart patient experiences in this early phase of treatment sets a definite tone for subsequent adjustment and rehabilitation. Data assembled by Klein and his associates (1965) suggests that one factor associated with myocardial infarction invalidism, namely fear of sudden death, has its origins in how patients and their spouses perceive and respond to their physicians' initial description of the illness. Finlayson and McEwen (1977:169) have observed that the onset of the heart attack itself "temporarily removes from patients the ability to make meaningful definitions of their individual situations and prospects; into this vacuum new and confusing definitions rush"; and Dominian and Dobson (1969:795) argue that "it is likely that the foundation of the individual's pattern of reaction is laid down when his anxiety and fears are at their greatest – that is, at the earliest stage of his illness."

The concepts of career and definition of the situation direct our attention as well to the patient's significant others. The drama of recovery from heart attack is played out in a number of different settings, including the home. Not only are the patient's spouse and children affected, socially and emotionally, by the illness, but by their actions they have direct impact on the patient's ability successfully to carry out the treatment regimen. This reality is reflected in the statement of the World Health Organisation cited in Croog, Levine and Lurie (1968) that, "Even Neurotic individuals can adjust to severe cardiac impairment if they are constantly integrated in a strong, supportive, reasonable but not overprotective, healthy family structure which accepts and understands the illness." What this statement also implies, however, is that in order for a well-intentioned, strongly-knit family structure to function effectively in this matter, the members must understand what is involved. What family members see, hear, and feel during the hospitalization can be crucial in this, especially since, as Williams and Rice (1977:393) have observed, "How the family perceives the patient's physical status on the ICU can be incongruent with what is actually happening." Moreover, Finlayson and McEwen (1977) discovered in their longitudinal study of over seventy heart attack victims and their spouses that, by the end of hospitalization, it was usual for couples to hold discrepant views on fundamental issues of prognosis and life style adjustment. This chapter will present data with respect to how patients *and* members of their families defined the situation they were experiencing during the ICU phase. We will compare the two perspectives and demonstrate how differences are related to aspects of the ICU as a social organization.

Comparison of Situational Contexts: Family, Patient

A) Entering the System

Once the patient arrived at the Emergency Room, he was separated from spouse, children, and friends, who waited for word of his fate in the busy hospital lobby. Family members were not permitted into the treatment area, although some tried to gain access surreptitiously. One wife told me that she tried but was "Screamed at" by a nurse. Another thought that it was taking a long time for the doctor to come, so when she heard her husband call out in pain, she went to him. She stayed only briefly, however, because she was afraid of being detected by a staff member. It was here in the lobby that families learned the diagnosis of heart attack from a staff physician. The news was direct and brief, followed immediately by instructions that the spouse of the patient should go to the Admissions Office to fill out the necessary hospitalization forms. Family members were often shocked at being told the husband or father had suffered a heart attack and needed "intensive care." Characteristically, they did not immediately respond to what they had been told. Even if the patient had severe, prolonged chest pain, or had had an electrocardiogram taken by the family physician prior to coming to the hospital, which showed serious abnormalities, they still held on to the hope that after examination and treatment at the hospital, the patient would be sent home with medication and a prescription for bed rest. For example, one spouse commented,

> Dr B. told me: "Your husband had a heart attack." I was still hoping that it wasn't, because Dr M. [the family doctor who sent them to the hospital] said *possible* coronary. I thought they would just do tests and he would be all right. He said, "Your husband had a heart attack." Like, you know, this is it.

With very few exceptions, there were few questions asked of the physicians, who did not remain with the families longer than it took to convey the diagnosis and instruct the spouse to go to the Admissions Office to complete insurance forms. No other staff person was assigned to the family at this point. During the few moments that a physician was present, the family members seemed unable to express their feelings or ask questions. From what I could learn, the physicians did not probe for questions or offer any assistance. Only one family member of all those I interviewed was brought out of the lobby to a private space in the treatment area where she could "let it all out." This occured because the woman in this case gave vent to her emotions, and although the physician was disturbed by her behavior, he had to deal with it. Her report of this is as follows:

> I just lost control: "Not my husband, no, no, no!" It wouldn't sink in. He, the doctor, got a little upset that I . . . so he said come in. I sat and just let it all out. I said, "Will he be all right?" The doctor replied, "Well, you know, he is pretty serious." I asked [him] at this time, "Should I let my daughter and son know?" He said, "That is your decision."

Once inside the treatment area the woman was able to seek out other medical personnel for reassurance and advice. She continued,

Dr K. was there and I said, "Will he be all right?" He said, "Don't worry. He has had severe heart damage, but don't worry." I said, "Should I tell my married children?" He said, "By all means let your son know." Very, very, decisive.

She apparently achieved what she needed at that time: someone to console, reassure, and advise her.

The patient in the Emergency Room had a different set of experiences. The structure of the physical space he was in allowed the conscious patient access to information about his condition which was qualitatively different from what his family received. It also provided more support for his emotional state and provided specific cues for active behavior. One patient recalled for me his impression of the Emergency Room:

Drs K. and B. came in with their stethoscopes. Meantime, the nurse is taking the cardiogram. Another is putting the I.V. needle in my arm. They then brought me into Xray. Dr B. explained a few things. He said, "When you go upstairs listen to the nurses, we will be around. Tomorrow don't be afraid if you see about ten or twelve doctors discussing your case." I said, "I won't get excited." From the time I got into this place to the time I left, the rapport of the Emergency Room was fantastic.

For patients who were conscious when they arrived on the ICU, the orientation which began in the Emergency Room continued. The nurses took an informal and friendly tone. First names were exchanged and there were often attempts at humor. The interaction had the tone of a primary group, in contrast to the family's bureaucratic handling. In the course of placing the patient in bed and attaching him to the specialized equipment, nurses not only engaged conscious patients in light conversation about their families, jobs, travels, and so on, but also explained to them important elements of their new environment. For example, in the course of being attached to the overhead monitor, patients not infrequently noticed the red alarm light flash on. After some initial fright, it was explained by the nurses that the alarm was

set off by a detached wire, which was the result of the patient's
sudden movement. Patients could see monitoring screens of
others and in the course of any day observed alarm lights
flashing numerous times. They learned by this that in all but a
few instances the cause was some mechanical difficulty, not an
emergency. The warm, nurturing tone the nurses took, their
willingness to explain the procedures of the unit, including
imparting the information that the patient could expect to
remain on the ICU for only a few days, helped to put patients
at ease, and made it easier for the staff to handle them. In
addition, these admission procedures served to mitigate any
fears the patients had that they were dying.

For family members, their typical experience upon initial
exposure to the ICU was of a different character entirely. It
reinforced what had been suggested by the way they were
handled earlier and established them as outsiders. Coming
into the ICU for the first time, the family members I
observed typically paused at the nursing station, but usually
did not speak with the nurses there. More often, they scanned
the room and went directly to the bed. There, they might
grasp the patient's hand, or just gaze intently. Few words
were exchanged. In a few moments they left.

What did *not* happen is significant. There was no systematic routine for introducing the family to the unit. The
wife's experience offers a typical illustration:

> They said in the Emergency Room that they would call me
> when they take my husband upstairs, and I could see him
> for a couple of minutes. So when I came out of the
> Admitting Room and he's upstairs, they told me he's up in
> the Intensive Care, so I went up there and my husband is in
> bed and they had, what do you call it, a monitor . . . When I
> went up I looked around, and I didn't ask anybody because
> I saw him and I went right up to him . . . The doctor was
> right there by his bed too . . . He asked how do I feel. I said,
> "all right." We stayed for about five minutes . . . They
> gave me a booklet [in the Admissions Office] you know,
> with visiting hours . . . If they wanted to tell me something
> important they would tell me . . . He [a friend] brought me
> home. He wanted me to have dinner with them, you know,
> but I was too tired and I was upset.

As the example cited above demonstrates, the entry experience allayed no fears or anxieties for wives, children, and others concerned with the patient. On the contrary, after leaving the hospital, they might often as not be completely disoriented as to time and space. "Then I went out and got lost getting home, but I got home – shattered," is how one person put it.

The experience that the family had suggests that those whose responsibility it was to organize patient care considered family members to have nothing to contribute to the staff's understanding of the patient. On the contrary, it was clear that the family's presence in the unit was considered potentially disruptive of the controlled atmosphere fostered on the ICU. So in contrast to the personal attention that was used to control patient behavior, staff controlled families by excluding them. The initial experience also presented the clear message that family members had no claim on the medical or nursing staff for assistance regarding their own suffering. They had so far been given no explanation of what to expect, including who was in charge of the case, or whether the patient would survive this heart attack. To this point, the family members in the hospital had largely been guided by formal procedures: fill out forms, wait to be told what to do next.

B) Organization of Perspectives

When the family members returned to the hospital the same day, or the next morning, their roles as passive outsiders were repeatedly reaffirmed. The space provided for the family members seemed designed to reflect the low value placed on the family role. Outside the unit there were few amenities or comforts of any kind. A row of hard plastic chairs were crowded together with no place for a family group to speak privately together. Moreover, the waiting area was also used to store various pieces of hospital equipment. Immediately inside the ICU door, just a few feet from where the visitors sat, was the facility for disposing of bed pans. The prevailing odor was one of spray deodorant and human waste.

Very little information about what was transpiring inside the unit was systematically conveyed to the waiting families.

There were no formal conferences held or any time set aside for questioning of either physicians or nurses. In fact, chances of encountering a physician on the ICU were, for the families, not good. The attending physicians, who examined patients each day, did their work prior to the first family visiting session. Residents were more often than not away from the ICU, or were there because of some urgent medical need and, therefore, unavailable for any kind of extensive interaction with families.

Staff members, doctors and nurses, did not initiate communication with families, and the latter did not seem able to strive to achieve it. When asked in interviews why they didn't ask the nurses the questions they had on their minds, the reply often was that "They (the nurses) are too busy." One said it would be "unethical" for a nurse to tell a family member the patient's blood pressure. There was also the suggestion that some family members thought that the nurses would become punitive if upset by their questions, and, as one person put it, "I need them now."

It was rarely recorded that a spouse, child, or other relative was assertive during this period of care in terms of asking questions of staff, or in any other way insisting on being kept informed about the day-to-day developments in the care. Family members often spent long hours waiting outside the unit, never once putting a direct question to a doctor or a nurse. Or, if a question was raised, it generally was in response to some significant change in the patient's condition which they noticed themselves or were informed about by one of the nurses. Complications would be brought to the family's attention and this, in turn, would stimulate staff–family interaction. In situations where the course of events was uncomplicated from a medical standpoint, family members were not seen to initiate interaction with staff, and were generally unable to report in any detailed fashion about the medical management of the illness, or about how the illness would affect their lives in the future. Patients, on the other hand, were relatively more active in acquiring information, and were seen initiating a great deal more conversation with the staff. The following illustrates the passivity which typified most families:

E.S.:   When you were visiting your husband this week [in the ICU] did you speak to any of the doctors at all?

SPOUSE: No.

E.S.:   Have you wanted to?

SPOUSE: They told my husband, you know, that the X-rays had shown he has a massive heart block. They told him and he just told me, and I didn't feel that I had to go to the doctor – he wasn't there anyway – or to the nurses, because they gave all the information to my husband and he told me, so what else could I do, right?

A few moments later, the woman was asked what her husband had been told by the staff. She replied, "He don't know. They don't tell him anything. So we have to wait and see, right?" Another wife of a patient always responded "Yes" whenever asked in the interviews if she had any questions for the doctor. Yet she was unable to specify what these were. Finally, prompted by repeated queries as to the nature of the information she wanted from the doctor but was unable to ask, she said in frustration: "I don't know about the heart. I probably wouldn't understand if they told me." She claimed that she did not speak to any physician until the very last day of the ICU stay.

One spouse who did try to seek out the attending physician told me during my first interview with her:

Dr K., who is the resident doctor there, is a wonderful doctor and a wonderful person. I said to him: "What has happened to my husband? What is the diagnosis? What must I do after he comes home?" Dr K. said: "You call Dr A. [the attending physician assigned to her husband's case] and make an appointment, and he will stay and sit with you for one hour and tell you everything, what to do, what has happened. Have him have it in writing." But forget it . . . He has no time to see the family of the patient. He is too busy.

In an attempt to elicit information, some family members, as they had done earlier in the Emergency Room, resorted to

what they considered to be deviant paths. One son claimed he
"sneaked a look" at his father's chart, and on the basis of what
he learned felt relieved that his blood pressure was within
normal limits. A wife also "looked over her [the nurse's]
shoulder" to see what was written in the chart. More often
than not, this only served to confuse rather than enlighten.

Much of what the families learned about the nature of the
care the patient was receiving, however, was conveyed by
inference. The structure of the situation for patients also
created barriers to information, and skewed their perceptions
of the situation. But for the families, the limitations on their
access to the setting had a more severe impact on their ability
to interpret what was transpiring. This is at the heart of the
differences between families' and patients' definitions of the
situation.

From the vantage point of the family, there was little to be
seen that did not reinforce their pessimistic view of the
patient's condition, which was that his safety was dependent
upon continuous medical monitoring and complete bedrest.
Seen from the outside, the ICU was a place where patients
were being heroically saved from death by the miracle of
technology administered by a highly-trained and dedicated
staff. Nothing reinforced this view better than the medical
emergencies that from time to time occurred. Emergencies
served to reinforce a view of the patient as precariously
balanced between life and death. When asked later what
images came to mind thinking of the ICU, the cardiac arrest
emergency was almost always mentioned. These events were
particularly frightening for family members. When they
occurred they brought medical personnel rushing into the
unit from other parts of the hospital and created an atmosphere of tension and uncertainty for friends and relatives
which was not relieved until they learned either that it was not
their loved one, or that the patient had been revived. As the
following excerpt from an interview suggests, the experience
is profoundly upsetting.

E.S.:   In other words, you saw the ICU as a frightening
             place?
SPOUSE: Well, the first time, yes. Of course, even up to

now I don't like watching that scope. I was telling you about the light flashing and all that. There's a lot of things going on there, too; there are emergencies. That make you [pause] . . . In fact, the first day he went downstairs, my son and I were leaving the hospital. As we were getting out of the elevator a nurse came darting into the elevator with two big needles like I've never seen anything like it taped to a cart or something. She said, "Please don't move!" She made a motion to push us back into the elevator. She had an emergency on the sixth floor. That was frightening in itself. Knowing he was on the third was a big relief – that it wasn't your own. You know how you feel. You don't want to see anyone suffer. But it wasn't your own.

As other investigations of heart attack patients have noted, patients utilize the emergencies and the deteriorating conditions of other patients around them as testimony of their own *relative* well being (McEwen 1973).

When emergencies did occur inside the unit or when several patients required extensive nursing care at the same time, the nurses were forced to pay less attention to the more stable patients. Patients often recognized this and used it to assess their own seriousness in relation to others. For patients, emergencies created a situation in which routines that normally underscored the critical nature of the patients' conditions were suspended and patients saw signs of their own well being reflected in the deteriorating conditions of others. An example of this can be seen in the following statement by a patient:

[At first] I was scared to death . . . The pain stayed with me from the time I got in there until about 7 o'clock at night. I wondered when is this pain going to leave me, you know. But once I got over the pain I felt good and I had no qualms. I didn't worry too much because I seen others around me that were worse off than me, like that Joe, he's got to stay four or five weeks.

The same function was served by the medical para-
phernalia which was very visible inside the unit. The monitor
flashing above the patient's bedside was particularly difficult
for outsiders to get used to as patients did. People tried to
compare each day's pattern to the last, and more often than
not could take no solace from the light beam's constant course
across the screen. Some days it seemed erratic or too fast, or
different from the patient's across the room. When the red
alarm flashed, the families were always concerned. People ran
from the room in tears because of misinterpreting the
monitor.

On the other hand, what was not visible to the families were
the various routines that were a normal part of everyday life
for the patients. Nor were outsiders attuned to the small
changes in the patient's care which coincided with improved
coronary functioning. Instead of being bouyed by seeing the
patient perform some small activity such as sitting outside the
bed, or shaving, family members were often puzzled and
apprehensive. It was difficult for families to accept the
freedom of mobility the patients gradually acquired since it
had not been explained to them and since their view of the
patient's condition was that any amount of strain or stress
could provoke injury. During family visiting, patients were
counselled by their spouses and children about the virtues of
obeying medical orders, especially those having to do with
remaining quietly in bed, and the vices of physical or mental
strain.

Patient–Family Differences in Defining the Situation

The separation of patient and family into different worlds of
experience was enforced for the entire length of the ICU stay.
Events which occurred regularly and in a variety of contexts
for the patients were observed only infrequently, if at all, by
family members, who were actually inside the unit for very
short periods of time. Interpretations which were made
reflected that portion of the process that was most clearly
evident to the patient and his family. While it is not possible
to account for all the difference between patients' and
families' definitions of the situation, some of what was
observed can be attributed to differential exposure to the day-

to-day occurrences that go on in and around the ICU. Let us now identify the major differences in the perspectives of patients and family members.

Throughout the stay, family members appeared more fearful and anxious than did the patients themselves, and in various ways gave evidence of a decidedly more pessimistic outlook for the future. One reflection of this pessimism can be seen in the fact that the possibility of the patient's death was more frequently mentioned or alluded to by family members than by patients. Interviewing family members was often made difficult by the overall emotionality of their responses. In contrast, patients were more even in describing what had and was occurring. It was rare for family members to joke about what they had seen or heard at the hospital, for example, but not so for patients. One of the more striking contrasts was in outlook for the future. In describing what the heart attack might mean to them in terms of their future lifestyles, wives and children invariably mentioned the significant alterations that would have to be made, frequently singling out jobs as a major area of change. Patients, in contrast, usually predicted a future in which little would change.

No doubt related to the above differences in response was the difference in the perception of healing. When asked any particular day whether their husbands seemed better, wives' answers emphasized the dangers that remained. In answering similar questions, patients, while not ignoring the critical nature of their condition, were decidedly more positive. Furthermore, wives' and children's views of the patients' conditions remained static throughout the ICU stay. An obvious manifestation of this inability to apprehend meaningful changes in the patients' state of health were the feelings the family members expressed about the patients' transfer from the ICU to another, less controlled, room in the hospital. They maintained, almost without exception, that the patient would be better off if he remained in the ICU for a while longer. Typical responses to questions that elicited feelings about transfer included the following:

Well, I think it would have been better [if the patient had remained on the ICU]. I mean, to stay on the safe side, although the doctor said that he was able to go down, because of the care that he was getting . . . They're very nice, you know. They were checking his blood pressure a couple times a day . . . They were taking his blood tests a couple times a day.

Another was: "I would feel it was good [to remain on the ICU] because they're right there for everything and there would be a lot more rest added to it."

Patients' reactions to being told they were leaving the ICU were significantly different. There was apprehension, to be sure, but the general response indicated that they interpreted the move as a positive development in the course of their treatment and a sign that they were getting better. The following patient's description illustrates his eagerness to leave the ICU:

Dr F. checked me over. He said, "You sound good. We're going to try to get you down there as soon as possible." I didn't know whether that meant that morning, in the afternoon, or the next day. Then the nurse came over . . . She wanted a urine specimen and she came back after an hour. She said, "Not yet?" I said, "No." She said, "Well you can go downstairs after you give me a specimen." So I said, "I didn't know *that*" [his emphasis], and with that I drew the curtains, and gave her the specimen.

Another element which typified the family's perspective was the failure to develop a clear understanding of what treatment consisted of, especially those activities that the patients undertook at the advice of the staff which were necessary for building strength and endurance. In short, family members thought it best that the patients have as little activity as possible; they equated activity with stress, repose with safety. In actual fact, patients were instructed by the staff of doctors and nurses gradually to begin certain kinds of activity, such as getting in and out of bed, moving limbs, and dangling their legs over the side of the bed. One could see in their behavior inside the unit, which was confirmed in speaking with them outside, that spouses and children tended to discourage patients from exercising even the small amount of freedom the unit allowed. This could be seen in the behavior of family members who urged patients to return to bed if they were seated in their chairs at the start of visitation. They responded the same way to other things the patients did, as in the case of a wife who tried to stop her husband from putting on his socks as he sat beside the bed. He was permitted out of bed and he was allowed to put on his socks. I observed one wife counselling the patient not to eat all of the food and use all of the condiments on his tray. She succeeded. Another patient was fed by a relative after being told he *could* and *should* feed himself. Although patients were often reluctant to perform many of these activities themselves, they did perform them and thus developed a perspective on activity that was different from that held by their wives and children.

It is significant to point out that the discrepancy which these behaviors represented was not a subject of discussion when families visited patients. As mentioned, visiting time was very brief. More to the point, however, in keeping with their perception of patients as highly fragile and easily susceptible to relapse if disturbed, family members deliberately refrained from discussing any topics directly related to the illness or treatment with the patient. The general approach was articulated by one spouse of a patient this way, "We didn't talk much to him while he was there, and likewise he to us. Because it was too much. We felt it would be better if he slept and rested." For some people, visiting was emotionally draining. They reported having all they could do not to burst into tears as they looked at their loved one who, all the time he was a patient on the ICU, was classified as "in critical condition." To the extent that spouse, child, and patient were aware of these differences, the cause was attributed to the other person's judgement, not to the different opportunities for observing and learning provided by the situation. Thus, spouses spoke of their patient-husbands as denying the full extent of their medical problem, or lacking proper caution and judgment. Patients, for their part, when this issue occasionally came up in conversation, attributed their wives' attitudes to "female worry" or lack of ability to analyze the problem correctly. The result was that issues like these went unaddressed, and were left for another time.

In sum, by the time of transfer to another part of the hospital, patients perceived their medical conditions as less threatening, appeared less worried, were more optimistic, and were better able to articulate a rationale for what was occuring than their families. Their attitudes toward their recovery were more positive and included a different, less fearful, view of physical activity.

To review, the first thing that occurred upon entry into the health care system was the separation of patient from his family. Undoubtedly based on a desire to isolate and treat the disease process and, at the same time, to avoid potentially disruptive external interference, the result was an abrupt rending of the family's social fabric and an assignment of the individuals needing help to passive, dependent roles. As so often happens where this occurs in delivering health care, there were unintended negative sequelae of a variety of types. We saw that the limitations placed on patient–family interaction did not stop family members from participating in the care process. However, because the family's interventions were based on an understanding of the situation which the patients did not share, the net effect was to create a barrier between patient and family, making visiting a source of stress rather than comfort for all parties. Also, since the viewpoint upon which family members based their actions in counseling the patients was also not shared by the staff, the result was the inverse of what the visitation policy was supposed to accomplish, which was family non-interference in patient care matters. Other authors (Minckley 1979) have suggested that families can have an upsetting effect on patients. Yet, our observation suggests that the reason this may be so is the failure on the part of the health care providers to incorporate the family members into the therapeutic process by informing them of all the relevant facts concerning the illness and the treatment and familiarizing them with the function of all modalities of therapy, including machinery, probing them for areas of uncertainty and concern, thereby stimulating their questions. An additional negative consequence was a lost opportunity for tapping the family's rich source of information about the patient which may have been useful to the caregivers. As Litwak and Meyer (1966) point out, members of primary groups share a knowledge of each other which is beyond the scope of a bureaucracy to obtain. Family members are intimately acquainted with how each responds to stress and what may comfort in such times. Yet, in attempting to relieve patients' stress, to comfort them, and to gather personal data of a sensitive nature, the health care system did not use the family members as informants in these matters, a role that a family member is eminently qualified to play.

The Patient's View of His Condition

It is important to examine the patient perspective on ICU treatment more closely in order that the picture we are presenting not appear distorted. In contrast with his family, the patient was, as stated, less fearful of the ICU environment. Yet, when looked at outside this context, patients exhibited considerable anxiety, particularly in the area of physical activity.

Anyone being treated in an intensive care unit for a heart attack is likely to be worried. The patient who is not is a special concern to the staff who are aware that denial of the realities of the situation may lead a patient to disregard medical advice, and do himself harm.

The ICU's routines appeared to be designed to relieve patients of the fear that they would die, not that they were not critically ill. In fact, as will be detailed below, much of what was said and done by the staff emphasized the seriousness of the illness. But staff actions seemed designed also to convince the patient of the importance of following instructions to the letter. In this way, staff sought to calm the new patient by convincing him that his death was not imminent; and keep him compliant by impressing him with the notion that his well being was contingent upon following orders. Invariably, the first order to the patient was to remain as immobile as possible. This included no unnecessary movement of body or limbs, no crossing of legs, no reaching. Patients were also told to call the nurses for any needs they had, and to follow all instructions they were given.

According to the view of the nurses at Group Hospital's

ICU, patients who were not worried about their condition were more likely to overstep the narrow boundaries set on their behavior, thus making their illness worse, than were those who exhibited concern. Most heart patients, I was told, begin to feel better after a couple of days rest and medication, and are alert even though they are still considered critical, and at risk for arrythmia. Emergencies brought on by patient overconfidence and resultant overactivity were cited by the nurses as one of the more serious problems of patient care they had to deal with. ICU staff nurses felt accountable for patients even after they left the unit. Deaths of patients on the General Medical Ward who had recently been cared for on the ICU were very much a matter of concern to the ICU nurses, especially if deaths occured suddenly and unexpectedly. Staff considered many of these post-ICU deaths to be mainly the result of patients' lack of judgement on the ward, and assumed they had been overactive – something their ICU experience should have taught them to avoid. When staff discussed a post-ICU death, they usually reviewed how the patient had behaved on the unit, whether he had shown signs of overconfidence. They recalled how often the patient had to be reminded to take his illness seriously. If a patient who had shown proper concern suddenly died, this seemed to remind the nurses of the inherent uncertainty of heart attacks.

As a way of controlling patient behavior, nurses often reminded the patients of the seriousness of their condition. Admonitions not to move in bed were often accompanied by statements like, "When you are critical you can't cross your legs." The "unworried patient" received singular attention. One day, speaking about a new patient who appeared to the staff to be taking his situation lightly (he was joking about it), and who had already been told of its seriousness, a nurse said to me, "I'd like to tell him what happened to Mr X [a former ICU patient who died on the General Medical Ward from a cardiac arrest] who acted just like he is now." On another occasion, a nurse-supervisor filling in on the ICU was speaking to a patient while making his bed. This patient had been admitted the day before in an unconscious state. He now appeared cheerful and remarked that when he came to the emergency room "for a few chest pains" he never expected to wind up in the ICU. The nurse asked if he remembered what had happened to him the first day of the unit. The man said that he didn't remember. She then wheeled to his bed a defibrillator (used in emergencies to deliver an electric current to the heart to correct a dangerous rhythm). She told him that this had been used to revive him and explained what the machine did. Speaking with me moments afterward, she said that it was good for patients to understand the threat of their illness.

It has been pointed out that, on Group Hospital's ICU there were no permanently assigned physicians. Outside of morning medical rounds, doctors appeared on the ICU usually only after being summoned by a nurse. This gave the nursing staff considerable responsibility for noticing the early warning signs of arrhythmias and cardiac arrest, and to respond immediately to treat the failing patient. A great deal of medical care was either carried out directly by nurses or initiated by them. They could not depend on physicians who were in other parts of the hospital.

The fact that patient survival was dependent to a degree on the performance of the nurses appears to have reinforced concern among the staff of the importance of restricting the patients activity and to define this as a primary part of their duties. Their belief that even cooperative patients could unwittingly precipitate a coronary event was used in explaining the need to never let the patient forget how fragile he was.

Patients knew from many sources that they were not supposed to exert themselves at all until they were otherwise instructed and were to ask the nurses when they needed anything, or wanted to move. Mr Warren explained to me:

> I was very shy up there, and very withdrawn. I waited until the last minute to ask them anything, rather than think I was disturbing them or making a nuisance of myself, you know. Although they hammer it into you: "Don't do anything for yourself. We are here to help you; just call and we will be there."

Patients who tried to do small things themselves and did not depend on the nurses were reprimanded. Mr Polski said he "caught hell" when he reached for an item on his bedside

table. He said he always tried to "help them" but "they won't
let me." Most patients were able to recall an incident where
they were corrected and reminded that the staff believed they
were in a very fragile state.

While nurses regularly corrected patients who did too
much it was rare to hear a patient be told he was not doing
enough. After being on the unit for a few days, patients were
instructed to do certain activities for a brief period of time,
such as sitting on the side of the bed "dangling," sitting in a
bedside chair, moving arms and legs. Later, they would be
allowed to wash and shave themselves.

Patients told me, and I observed, that they often tended to
do *less* than they were allowed to. More than once while I was
with Mr Ambrosio, he returned to bed before his allowable
time out of bed was up. Once he told me, "I don't want to
overdo it, they were great to let me up." Another patient
returned to bed because he wanted to "save up" his time for
visitors. Mr Goldberg's approach to activity on the ICU was:
"The more rest I get here, the quicker I get back to normal at
home." When patients did not do as much as they were
allowed, the nurses did not seem to take notice of this, at least
they acted as if they didn't notice. There were exceptions.
One involved a patient who refused to wash, shave, or feed
himself. His consistent, almost total, inactivity resulted in a
staff initiated psychiatric consult. In general however, as long
as a patient did some part of the activity that was asked of him,
he could expect not to have any difficulties with the nurses.
Doing less than one was allowed to seemed to derive from the
high value placed on immobility and dependency. In addition
to being suspicious and afraid of activity, patients seemed to
draw an inference that doing a little less than allowed could
actually *aid* the recovery process. The virtues of controlled
mobility which, according to medical sources is an integral
component of ICU treatment, were much less visible to
patients than were the potential negative results of over
activity.

These circumstances fostered the attitude that activity
should be undertaken very cautiously. I suspect that without
the close proximity of the nurses, some patients would have
done less than they actually did do. But because they were

watched so closely, and did want to be "good patients", a
certain amount of ritual compliance was the result. However,
the underlying attitudes, fears, and perceptions of patients
toward their illnesses which led them to want to do less than
the situation actually called for, rarely became exposed as
issues of care to be responded to by the medical staff.

The medical equipment on the unit aided nurses in
detecting patients' activity. Movement of a patient could
dislodge the lead to the monitor causing the alarm light to
flash the news to the nurse who would respond by correcting
the patient. Activity that caused the heart rate to increase also
tripped the warning device. Blood pressure readings, done
frequently during the day, could also indicate if the patient
had been too active. I learned this in a very personal way.
Shortly after I interviewed Mr Polski for the first time on the
ICU, a nurse took his blood pressure and announced to me
that the interview had caused the patient's pressure to rise.
"That's the most activity he's had since he's been here" she
said. There were no equivalent aides to identify *inactivity*.

There are, of course, patients who feel that their conditions
do not warrant the kind of restrictions the ICU placed on
them. Mr Polski is an example. Mr O'Shea, who exclaimed in
an interview, "I still can't believe I had a heart attack," is
another. Yet the vigilance of nursing staff succeeded in
keeping patients such as these two from acting out their
deviant opinions.

Patients typically asked few questions about the condition
of their health, about the progress of the therapy, or of what to
expect when they left the unit. Mr Asti said, "I tried not to
show curiosity," and his characterization of his interaction
with medical staff was that he took the "ostrich approach."
His bed was closest to the nursing station, perhaps five feet
away. Yet he said he engaged in no conversation at all, and
even tried not to listen in on their conversation. Mr Ambrosio
said, "Since I have been here I have never asked anyone –
doctor, nurse, or resident – what happened, how is the heart,
what happened and how is it improving." With medications,
he took the same approach, "Here is the medicine, down the
hatch . . . I never would say what is the green pill, or the
yellow pill, or the blue pill, whatever it was. I never asked any

questions." He summed up his philosophy this way: "My whole concept since the day I came here was: Don't worry. Let your mind go blank."

A similar approach was expressed by another patient, Mr Goldberg. This was a man in his early sixties who had complained of chest pains for weeks before his attack. He then was given nitroglycerine by his physician, a fact that Mr and Mrs Goldberg used in arguing after the attack that if their family physician had hospitalized him sooner, the coronary might have been prevented. He told me he asked few questions in the ICU because, "If they want me to know something important, they'll tell me." However, he also revealed that he was frightened of what he might learn from questioning staff members. He said, "If you question too much, he'll make a slip he doesn't mean." Fear of having bad news was expressed by other patients. For example, Mr Ambrosio told me: "If you ask questions, they're under pressure. They don't want to be in a position of saying 101 per cent that you will be alive."

Other patients reported not inquiring about the details of their treatment because they "knew" they wouldn't be told. Moreover, they seemed to indicate that they had no right to this information. Mr O'Shea said it would be "unethical" for a staff person even to tell him what his blood pressure reading was. Mr Grasso similarly offered that it was the doctor's prerogative whether to reveal information to him or not.

Questioning was, in a number of ways, discouraged. On morning rounds the medical director led a review and discussion of each patient's progress with eight to ten medical residents and the nurses. This occurred at the bedside of each patient. In effect, the patient's present state of health was analyzed: his latest ECGs were analyzed for changes in pattern, lab reports were reviewed. The discussion was highly technical with no effort made to translate into lay terms for the patient. Without having knowledge of the technical language, patients could not participate during rounds. Patients were told they "should not be concerned" with the proceedings, and the way doctors explained this event to the patients implied that rounds had little relevance to them. Mr O'Shea told me he was forewarned in the emergency room that in the morning a group of doctors would examine him but "Don't worry about it, it involves medical stuff. It's academic so don't let it perturb you." New patients were almost always told by the medical director that what was being discussed was "for the doctors," and they "should not be disturbed" by the discussion or by the fact that ten doctors were examining them. What he seemed to be implying was: "Your condition is not your concern." Patients on the unit for several days were also sometimes reminded not to take too great an interest in rounds. One morning after Mr Goldberg's care had been discussed at his bedside, the medical director told him "not to mind" what had just transpired. Later, Mr Goldberg told me he should have replied that he was "listening to further my medical studies" which was a rather incisive bit of humor. I asked what he had heard that morning. He replied, "technical jargon." Did he ask any questions at the time? "No."

Generally, no questions were asked of the patient at rounds that allowed any expression of his opinions or feelings. Questions asked required only a yes or no answer, as when the patient is asked: "Do you get a pain when I touch you here?" The few patients I observed who did expand statements of how they felt, or who tried to inquire why they felt pain or continuing discomfort were either given very brief responses to their statements or were interrupted by the medical director who told the resident to explain to the group the details of the case.

Even the positioning of the staff vis-a-vis the patient constrained against his participating in discussions of his own case. During the proceedings, the medical director stood behind each patient and spoke out to the residents and nurses who were gathered around the body – sometimes looking at long ECG print outs strewn across the patient's body which was used like a table for lab reports, charts, and ECG print outs. To address the medical director, the patient would have to turn around, a movement that was not permitted.

Before the group moved to the next patient, the director usually – although not always – made a statement to the patient that he "was doing fine," or "the best thing you can do for yourself now is take it easy." I never heard him tell a patient he was not doing well. Usually something positive was said. Patients acted passive; by far the most frequent statements made by patients during rounds were in response to humorous remarks to them from the medical staff. They seemed pleased when doctors joked with them.

Events Preceding Transferring the Patient to the General Medical Ward

Another factor which may have had a bearing on why patients did not raise issues or questions they had about their illness, their progress, or their future care was the time orientation of the unit, which emphasized the present. The unit had only two small windows and these gave little natural light. The room, dim at all times, made it appear as if time were not moving. Patients often remarked that they were unaware of the time or that they were surprised when they found out the time of day.

As the time of transfer to the General Medical Ward approached, the condition of the patient was expected by the staff to have changed for the better. On the ward he would not be monitored electronically, and nurses would be less available to observe him closely. Also, a patient would be given more personal choice over his own movements. On the ICU there were no organized procedures to prepare a patient for this change. There was little discussion of what was in store in the future. There were few opportunities for patients to anticipate the future and raise questions about the state of their health.

In many ways patients about to be transferred off the unit were treated just as they had been as newly arrived patients. Restrictions on activity remained severe up until transfer. All patients, new and old, spent most of the day in bed. Time out of bed sitting in a chair was brief, walking was almost non existent. Even in cases when patients were allowed to sit out of bed at will, they generally spent most of the time in bed. All patients, new or old, were attached to the monitor. Schedules were the same, as were visiting regulations. To the end, the emphasis was on what the patient should *not* do.

Patients had little advance warning as to the time of their

transfer off the ICU to the General Medical Ward. Even a patient who felt better and who had been allowed to sit out of bed could not be sure when he would leave. Mr Warren told me: "They'd rather keep you here as long as they can, because you have all them gadgets on you and they can keep better tabs on you."

Mr Asti was told during the morning rounds that he would be leaving the unit. Less than three hours later he was transferred.

As previously stated, patients were given an estimate of their probable length of stay soon after their admission into the ICU. But they were also told at that time, and if they asked again, that the exact timing of the transfer depended upon a bed being available for them on the General Medical Ward. So when they were told they were leaving, it came as a surprise, and they had little time to make the adjustment.

After patients are told they would be transferred, they received instructions that were similar to those they had been receiving all along: do not be active, be cautious. The statement, "Take it easy down there; no running around. We don't want to see you back up here," was repeated with slight variation each time a patient left. Mr Ambrosio said he was told: "Some people . . . They think they can go back and feel like Superman. But that is where they make their mistake."

Until they leave the ICU, patients were constantly reminded of their fragile physical conditions. They were continually treated by means that emphasized their dependency on the nurses and the life support technology. Symbols that indicated progress were few in comparison with those indicating statis.

The Intensive Care Unit is not only a setting for the care of the seriously ill, but it is also a point of entry into a system of health care. The experiences the patients and their families had suggests that these two functions are not easily blended. Being on the ICU constrained against anticipating the next level of care, or appreciating what changes had taken place in health status. The day-to-day routines minimized the patients' awareness of their own physical integrity, discouraged questioning or anticipating problems to be faced once the rigid restraints against mobility were lifted. These

same structural factors also prevented the family of the
patient from expressing and staff from noticing and/or
dealing with fears, uncertainties, and misunderstandings. In
the following section, we will deal with the consequences of
such lack of socialization into the health care system.

Becoming Non-Critical

Patients went directly to the General Medical Ward from the
ICU. In this new care setting the recovering heart patients
were placed side by side with those who either had been on
the ICU earlier, or had other illnesses. The physical conditions of the roommates varied considerably. Some newly
arrived post-ICU patients were placed in rooms with men
considered by the nurses to be dying. In other cases, their
roommates were active and about to go home.

As soon as the patients arrived on the ward, they become
virtually indistinguishable from other non-coronary patients.
There were no oscilliscopes monitoring the heart rate, nor
nurses observing them. All were given permission for some
ambulation and could use the bedside commode or walk to
the toilet if there was one inside the room. Their schedule
of meals and other routines were identical with non-
coronary patients.

Considering the restraints these patients had been under
up to the moment of their transfer, the situation they now
found themselves in represented a considerable shift in
emphasis. Mr Asti recalled that when he arrived in his room
on the ward the only instructions he received were "not to
leave the room, don't wander." He suddenly had choices he
didn't have before; just as when he arrived on the ICU his
options had been suddenly and drastically reduced. Each
setting had its own structural constraints which the patient
had to adjust to.

To some patients the lifting of restraints posed a dilemma.
Their self definition as seriously ill patients which was
fostered and nurtured in the ICU seemed incompatible with
the less restrictive climate on the ward, and threatened their
sense of security. Patients who felt they still needed to have
medical expertise in close proximity to themselves as was the

case moments earlier were suddenly faced with the prospect that they "were now on their own."

One typical mode of patient adaptation to the General Medical Ward was to continue behaving as if one were still on the ICU. In spite of the greater opportunities for autonomy and freedom of movement some patients remained committed to the values and norms of the ICU. I asked Mr Asti, who arrived on the ward at about 11.00 am, when he first met any of the medical staff. He recalled that a "nurses' aide" came in during the afternoon with medication, and at about four a nurse gave him an injection. Even though he was told only not to wander out of the room, he did not walk in the room at all; he continued to sit next to his bed or was in the bed all day. He remained passive and inactive, in accordance with his self image as a seriously ill patient.

Mr Ambrosio is a case example of a patient committed to his ICU perspective who attempted to impose his own definition onto the staff. I was present during his first interaction with a ward nurse. He had been waiting anxiously for one of the medical staff to arrive, and was disturbed that this did not occur immediately. When the nurse came to the bedside she asked his name and seemed to check it against her notes. She asked if he had been given instructions from his physician, and when Mr Ambrosio indicated that he had, she began to back away toward the door still jotting notes. Mr Ambrosio began to speak rapidly, saying that he was told on the ICU to restrict his movements to the area between his bed and the near wall. He moved to the end of his bed and drew an imaginary boundary line with his finger. He seemed to be trying to slow the nurse's departure, to inform her of all the instructions he had been given – not to overtire himself, to walk a little but sit or go to bed when he felt he was tiring. She didn't reply verbally, but nodded her head and left the room. Within a half hour an aide brought him his lunch. She placed the tray several feet from his bed, beyond the boundary line he had earlier drawn. He would not retrieve it. Later, when a nurse noticed the tray she asked Mr Ambrosio why he had not eaten. He told her that his doctor did not allow him to walk the distance required to get the tray. Later he told me he was glad this had happened because it gave him the opportunity to convey to the nurses what his regimen was supposed to be.

For patients like Mr Asti and Mr Ambrosio the sudden shift in the orientation of the medical staff came unexpectedly. They behaved in a manner that suggested that they were frightened of no longer being under the scrutiny of medical experts, that they were not confident of their ability to act on their own. Although the structure of the General Medical Ward allowed patients the freedom to increase their mobility and expand their level of activity, the manner in which patients were suddenly moved there from a setting that demanded passivity and caution served actually to increase their psychological dependency. In the absence of medical personnel insisting on inactivity and dependency, some patients demanded this of themselves as a defense against the dangers of over confidence which had been internalized during their ICU stay. At least at the outset the General Medical Ward routines had, for some patients, an effect that was the opposite of that which was intended.

Not all patients, however, were disturbed by the absence of restrictions and staff to enforce them. To some the ward provided freedom of movement they wanted but could not obtain on the ICU. Mr Polski immediately left his room and walked through the corridors, even though he was told "not to wander" from his room. Mr O'Shea did the same. Both believed that the hospital's routines were generally too harsh for their own cases, and took advantage of the relative lack of nursing contact on the ward to expand their activities.

Regardless of the definition a patient held of his condition as he entered the ward, he could find evidence to reinforce his perspective.

3

The Hospital Experience Continued: Toward Homecoming

In its design, the General Medical Ward had the potential for greater family access both to patients and to staff than the ICU had. Visiting hours extended from before noon until eight in the evening. Unlike the ICU setting, the ward did not have the same spatial and bureaucratic barriers between staff and visitors; doctors, nurses, patients, and visitors all shared the same space. In the way that the space was arranged, doctors and nurses were visible as they worked in and around the patients' rooms. The nurses' station was not out of bounds to visitors as it had been on the ICU. At any time during the long visiting period, family members could have approached the station and questioned the nurses directly. Yet, in most instances, this did not happen. Little more family–medical staff interactions took place on the ward than was the case on the ICU. As a consequence, the concerns, doubts, and misconceptions about the treatment process which we observed on the ICU continued unabated, and even increased among the family members right up until the time of hospital discharge.

For the families the ICU had a "halo effect," and like the patients they used what they had seen to be the procedures there to interpret what was now occurring on the ward. Many family members questioned the lack of official sanctions against patient activity, and continued to persuade the patients to remain sedentary. At times they blamed the ward staff for not enforcing a stricter regimen and were critical that the nurses were not around the patient as much as ICU nurses were. Mrs O'Shea, for example, claimed that the nurses allowed her husband to do things on his own because they were "lazy" and "they take advantage of his good nature."

She told me that when she visited, "I was the nurse when I was here." Since she presumed he was out of bed often while she was not present, when she arrived to visit she ordered him into bed. In an attempt to reduce his walking, which he was permitted by the staff to do within the room until he was tired, Mrs O'Shea refused to bring him his pajamas or robe from home. He was left with only the hospital robe which was open in the back and which Mr O'Shea felt embarrassed to be seen in. When he was sent back to the ICU, his wife told me she was pleased.

It is not difficult to understand why the ICU had such a "halo effect" on the families. The strategy for dealing with the illness on the ICU seemed like "a sure thing." The men had entered the unit under a threat of death and were still alive. People had witnessed that the ICU could efficiently cope with emergencies; in contrast the efficiency and protective ability of the ward was an unknown commodity and from the perspective of many family members it left something to be desired.

In addition to being upset because the ward staff seemed to take a casual, and in the family's view, inappropriate stance toward patient care, wives told me that they were worried that the staff was not placing adequate controls on what patients learned of their conditions. Mrs Grasso said:

> They speak very frank to them. They come right out and tell them everything. I've been able to get quite a bit of information from Tony. Here is one thing I have to say which left me a little bewildered. One of the doctors, not our family doctor, some doctor had said to him, "People who have heart attacks would have had them anyway no matter what they did." And then in the second vein they tell you not to smoke. Not to over-eat, you know, be careful. Now how do they expect a patient who is coming home to start a new life to worry about what they are going to do if they have that in the back of their minds that they're going to get a heart attack anyway?

Mrs Grasso was troubled that her husband would not tolerate a strict regimen if he did not believe it would bring complete recovery. In effect, she was accusing the medical staff of abandoning its culturally sanctioned charge that nurses and doctors are expected to work for full recovery from illness. Mrs Grasso, however, did not confront the staff directly with her complaint. Instead she took upon herself the responsibility of convincing her husband that full compliance with a strict interpretation of the medical regimen would make him well.

Mrs Stein also came to doubt the judgement of the staff. She told me that she could "wring the neck of that doctor who told him it was OK to smoke a couple of cigarettes a day." Mrs Ambrosio was fearful that if the doctor told her husband what he told her, it would cause her husband to lose his will to do everything possible to get well. The doctor told her that her husband would never again be able to do anything as strenuous as changing an automobile tire. When I asked her if she relayed this information to her husband she replied: "If I tell him that in the future you can't do this or that, he will say: 'What the heck, I'd rather not get better.' I'm afraid of that." Her response was similar to Mrs Grasso's. She emphasized to her husband that full compliance with a strict interpretation of the medical regimen was the only way to recovery.

The wives felt that it was important for the patient to believe he would eventually recover fully, even if they themselves believed this to be unrealistic. In this way, they reasoned, the patients would not balk at restrictions on their behavior. Staff members who were "realistic" in discussing the illness and its probable consequences with the patients were considered by the wives to be exercising rather poor judgement.

We can see that the wives questioned the approach to care taken on the ward. They preferred the care on the ICU where patients were allowed no discretion, and where the patients seemed very secure because every action was taken under medical supervision. In effect, when the wives visited, they attempted to recreate the atmosphere of the ICU, since they could not count on the ward medical staff to do so. The discrepancy between the wives' definition of the situation and their perception of staff behavior created a barrier to wife–staff communication. The wives felt they had to make up for the failure of the staff to impose strict restraints against patients doing too much.

The ward offered no incentives to give up the first

impression. The family members continued to believe that any benefits which might be expected to accrue from activity were small when compared with the potential dangers.

Awareness that it was good for patients to have an active orientation was almost non existent. They continued the practice begun in the ICU of negotiating with the patients to do less than they wanted to. Patients sometimes resisted their families on this and conflict could develop. One Strategy patients had of dealing with members of their families who continually tried to have them remain in bed, or not to talk too much, was to suggest that they visit less. It was common for a patient to urge his spouse to telephone rather than visit every day, or to reduce the actual length of the visits. Sometimes spouses did reduce their visiting time when the differences between them and the patient were beginning to become apparent.

There was, in general, little interaction between patients and the members of their families about the details of the care or of the kind of adjustments that would have to be made in the lives of the family members after hospitalization. Again the absence of conflict was a sign of failing to discuss different points of view rather than consensus over issues of concern of the parties. Family members continued to be worried about potential harmful effects of open discussion and avoided many topics. Mrs Grasso, for example, noticed that her husband seemed to be receiving intravenous medication. I asked if she inquired of him what it was for. She replied that she "didn't want to press it. I didn't want to speak about it too much." Mrs Ambrosio deliberately withheld certain kinds of information she learned about the illness for fear it would upset her husband.

Even when important topics concerning aspects of re-covery did come up, the conversation was likely to be shifted to more benign areas. This shift was especially likely to occur when the parties to the interaction realized that the issue raised was one on which there discrepant views. Mr O'Shea said that there were several times when he and his wife had to "bite their lips" so as not to become angry over something one of them said. When, for example, he spoke of returning to his job his wife would respond that he should not; but when he persisted with this theme she tried to change the subject, rather than argue with him. When she mentioned plans she had at home which he disagreed with (for example, how much money to spend on their daughter's wedding), he kept silent because "I don't want to get into a hassle with her." Normally, he said, he would have vigorously pressed his viewpoint regardless of how angry they both got.

Mr Grasso was often despondent in the hospital over what his chances were to hold a decent job once his recovery period was over. He was preoccupied with a fear that he would only be able to get a very menial position. I asked his wife if she discussed this problem with him:

Every so often he'll have the paper in front of him and he reads different kinds of want ads . . . One night he said: "I'll address envelopes at home." So you can see he's reading little things like that. And we change the subject, or laugh at him and tell him first one step at a time, first you get well and then take it one step at a time.

By tacit agreement, the spouses had no exchance of views, and areas of potential conflict were unexplored and remained dormant.

Adjusting to The Ward Routine

Left to decide on their own the pace of daily living on the ward, a number of patients took a highly conservative approach to their activities up to the time of their discharge. They never seemed to find a balance between caution and confidence but preferred to "stay on the safe side." Mr Warren told me shortly before he left the hospital that he had the "freedom of the room." I asked how active he actually was. He replied: "Mostly walking from here to the bathroom and back to the chair. You don't like pacing the floor or anything. I've either been in the chair or sitting like this in the bed. I'm trying to take it as easy as I can." Mr Asti took a very similar approach. He had exhibited a considerable amount of fear of activity since he entered the hospital. By the time of his discharge, these fears seemed to be unabated:

E.S.:   Did [the doctor's] telling you that you are leaving
           and here are the instructions make you a little more
           active?
Mr Asti: No, outside of walking across the room to get out of
           the way of people working, that was all.
E.S.:   And was it different the previous day?
Mr Asti: No.
E.S.:   Or the day before that?
Mr Asti: No.

On the other hand, some patients used what they saw or
experienced to justify engaging in desired behavior, some of
which was clearly in violation of hospital rules. Mr Stein, for
example, learned that not all staff members would express
serious opposition to patients' smoking in the hospital. He
was aware that other patients used the toilets in the hall to
smoke and that their behavior was not exposed to criticism.
He also learned that there were people who would supply
patients with cigarettes – visitors, even some aides. He told
me that while he was waiting to be given tests in the basement
lab area he asked a staff member for a puff on this person's
cigarette and this was granted. He began regularly to join the
other smokers in the bathrooms in the hall. He even smoked
in his own room, and claimed that some nurses detected this
but said nothing. He did receive a harsh criticism from a
nurse on two occasions, and stopped smoking in the room
when she was on duty. Being detected smoking by a nurse,
however, did not result in any more disciplinary action than
being told to stop. No one ever came to Mr Stein to discuss
his smoking even though he was detected. His own belief was
that several cigarettes a day would do him no harm – and he
could point to medical staff who by their tolerance of his
behavior seemed to support his viewpoint. By the time he left
the hospital, however, he said he had "failed completely" to
hold his smoking to only a few cigarettes a day.
   Mr Polski noted that the attention he received from nurses
had been diminishing steadily since he arrived on the ward.
For example, he said, "Now that my blood pressure is
normal, they don't take it half as much as they used to." Then
he related a story about a nurse who came into the room to

take patients' temperatures. She is alleged to have said: "Oh, you don't need it" and with a wave of her hand she dismissed his need for this procedure. This delighted him since it gave evidence for his point of view. He constantly sought out examples to reinforce a belief that in his case the routines of the hospital were too strict. As he had earlier, in the final days of his ICU stay, he made the judgement that the instructions given him were cautionary but not essential to his well being. He told me: "Lying here is not going to get me any stronger. That's why I try to do more every day." He began a daily program of exercise which he knew to be outside the general limits set by his physician. First he tested himself regularly to learn how much strain he could tolerate by lifting heavy objects around the ward, even though he did once feel a stab of chest pain. He started by lifting chairs and pushing heavy doors. He walked up and down the halls before he was even permitted out of the room. When I asked him if he thought this was advisable in his condition he replied that if he allowed himself to remain inactive he would not be strong enough later when he wanted to resume building his country home. To put his strengthening program into effect he learned when the nurses were changing shifts and their attention would be diverted.

We might examine the actions of these patients against the theoretical framework of the doctor–patient relationship suggested by Szasz and Hollender (1956). In their terms the recovery from an illness like heart attack would involve a progression of stages of the doctor–patient relationship. The first stage, *Activity–Passivity*, might characterize the most acute phase of the illness and be appropriate during ICU care. Here the orientation is one in which the patient is more or less completely helpless and the physician *does* something to him.

Once the patient is capable of following instructions and exercising some judgement, as the men on the General Medical Ward were expected to do, a new stage of the doctor–patient relationship – *Guidance–Cooperation* – is supposed to replace Activity–Passivity. As Szasz and Hollender (1956) explain, in this approach the patient is expected to look up to his physician and obey him. While the patient is still very much dependent on medical advice, the success of the therapy requires the patient to adopt the physician's goals as his own, and *act* on them. But, as we have seen, the patient might comply with certain directions because the doctor so *orders* and the staff enforces them, not because the patient himself understands and accepts the need for such a course of action. Another reason why the hospitalized heart patient may cooperate with the prescribed regimen may be because he feels reassured that the presence of medical experts will protect him from the harm that may accompany his increased activity. Without such reassurance the fearful patient might incline toward doing less than ordered.

Patient care routines on the General Medical Ward suggest that the staff took for granted that the *Guidance–Cooperation* mode of doctor–patient relationship was operative. However, for some patients the change in their care to less intense, frequent, and controlling staff involvement only imbedded more firmly them in a passive–dependent orientation, while other patients responded to the ward routines by becoming more self-initiated, and thus more active, than the staff expected. The organization of care at Group Hospital operated under the assumption that Activity–Passivity would prevail on the ICU and Guidance–Cooperation on the ward. The staff behaved according to these organizational expectations. The patients were led by these same organizational constraints either to continue their dependency, or to move beyond the expected level of self sufficiency.

The fact that the patients saw their attending physicians each morning did little to expose patients' deviant attitudes and behavior to the staff, or clarify the intentions of the physicians with regard to the purpose or content of the regimen. Patients gave information to physicians about the content of their daily activities in the same general terms as the physicians had used in describing the regimen. A patient might say, "I feel OK, I do some walking each day and when I get tired I sit down," and it would apply to a patient doing very little, just as well as to a patient doing quite a bit. They were not encouraged to elaborate. Patients like Goldberg and Asti who remained very sedentary on the ward because they were fearful of reinjury, could answer affirmatively when asked if they were getting on their feet. They had occasion to be active – walking to the bathroom, moving while the room was being cleaned, and other times when they were *forced* to move. Since the doctors did not specify the amount of exercise the men should take, or to what degree they should be increasing their activities, the men could believe they were, in general terms, compliant and could present themselves to their doctors as such. This general answer always seemed to satisfy the doctors who did not demand to know specifically what the patients had done or their reasoning behind it. Based on patient interviews, there was never any testing of patients' knowledge of the regimen, nor did it seem that questions from patients were encouraged except for those of the most basic type (i.e. Can I use the toilet in the hall?). Questions put to patients by doctors remained technical (Where did you feel the discomfort?). Patients did not seem to be encouraged to give more than very brief answers, often of the yes or no type. Patients like Mr Polski and Mr O'Shea who knew they were going beyond the bounds set by their physicians seemed able to convey that they were doing less than they actually were and to hide their activity. Mr Polski, who did not reveal to staff his activity program, said his doctor told him, "If all my patients had your attitude, my job would be half done." Mr Polski was cheerful when his doctor came, told him he felt good, and indicated he was accepting the hospital routine. Indeed, since he had figured out how to "beat the system" he was cheerful and had no complaints. Mr O'Shea was not reluctant to misinform staff. When a nurse asked if his doctor allowed him to be out of bed one morning after he had experienced pain the night before, he replied yes. When the nurse left, he turned to me and said he actually had been told to remain in bed for the day.

One wonders about the lack of probing questions asked by the staff to determine if patients understood the recovery process. Patients were certainly not revealing this information on their own. One must realize that the physicians assigned to patients at Group Hospitals would not be following up the case later during the home recovery period. Their focus was on the immediate medical situation, not on attitudes and perceptions that would have a bearing on the way patients responded to the medical regimen later on when they were no longer their responsibility. As long as there was no indication of any exacerbation of symptoms neither patients nor medical staff seemed to raise questions about compliance. If X-rays, electrocardiograms, and the other medical tests were within the normal limits, and the patients experienced no chest pain, everyone seemed satisfied. The patients were content to continue behaving in the future as they had in the recent past. For the sedentary ones this meant that their highly cautious response had been responsible for their present state of relative well-being and they were not motivated to change a strategy that seemed to work for them. On the other hand, active patients looked on their present progress as confirmation that their self-initiated activities were not harmful and might even have helped.

Toward Homecoming

Patients concerns and those of the families were for the most part centered on the hospital. Thoughts of home and the problems to be faced after hospital discharge were not at the forefront of awareness. When questions about post hospital care did surface, few people were active in seeking answers from staff. The absence of attention to the post-hospital period cannot be solely attributed to lack of initiative, denial, or short-sightedness on the part of patients and their close kin to matters that would begin to occupy them in an intense way in only a couple of weeks.

Much of what patients and families did or did not do about preparing themselves and their homes for the patients' return home was the result of how they interpreted certain policies and other messages from hospital personnel, and what the ward structure conveyed by implication.

Most of the patients and family members believed that it was hospital policy that shortly before the patient was discharged, they would be called to a meeting with several members of the staff – including physicians and dietitians – to be informed about home care. They were, in other words, aware of a certain timetable, medical care came first, receiving information about post-hospital roles and responsibilities was placed somewhere toward the end of hospitalization –

exactly when no one knew. My questions to Mrs Grasso on the topic of preparing for home care and her answers are very typical of the other spouses:

E.S.: Did the doctors say how long he would be in the hospital?

Mrs Grasso: They said as long as he keeps progressing, the beginning of next week.

E.S.: Did they say anything yet about what his life style would have to be like?

Mrs Grasso: No, they said when he's ready to leave they will prepare him for it; the diet, and what to do and not to do.

Near the end of the hospital stay I asked Mrs Warren: "So at this point you really don't know what his mobility will be?" She replied, "No, I don't, I would like to see one of the doctors, but I'll wait now until he comes home. And then see what he really can do."

Mr Ambrosio, however, was concerned about how he would manage at home, especially since he was told he would have to inject himself with insulin every day. When he expressed his concerns, his physician and nurse assured him that all of his questions would be answered some time later. Mr Ambrosio spoke with me about the schedule for preparing him for post-hospital care:

I told the head nurse: "You know its amazing that they have no booklets or literature on the subject. I don't want a medical dissertation on the subject, just plain, simple facts. What am I to do? Why, how and when? It is as simple as that." She said she would look into it. . . . Then I said [later to a doctor]: "Who gets the follow-up report? After I leave here what am I just number 45559, like a prison number?" He said "Before you leave you will get everything you need. The attending doctor will come in and will give you everything, and instruct you what to do, and what not to do."

In effect, the medical staff was conveying to patients and family members its particular order of priorities. First, the medical aspect of care are dealt with, and only then are rehabilitation issues addressed. Bloom (1965:116) argues that this two step process of establishing capability before teaching the patient to utilize his capability emerges from a hierarchy of values embedded in modern medical practice: "Especially within the rational, doing, future-oriented cultural frame of reference of Western society, reinforced by the marriage of science to medicine, the technical foundation step toward rehabilitation has been primary."

Patients had few resources with which to press any demands for information they may have had. Not many could take the direct approach of Mr Stein in dealing with staff. He told me that he had been impatient with his doctor who "kept his motor running" when he looked in on him. Mr Stein recalled the following incident. One day the doctor asked if he was having any pain. Mr Stein had had pain the night before and wanted to be sure to express it clearly so the doctor would realize it was a different kind of pain than he had been having previously. He paused to construct his answer but the doctor began to step away and Mr Stein thought he would leave before he could answer. So he lunged at the doctor and held him by the lapels of the jacket. Mr Stein then said to him if he wanted an answer he would have to wait a moment. Mr Stein reported that after this incident, his doctor seemed more patient and spent more time with him.

Another factor in why families and patients seemed to ask few questions about the outpatient home care period was that it was widely believed, incorrectly, that after the patient left the hospital the specialists encountered at the hospital would continue to control the care. In other words, it was perceived that there would be no break in the continuity of care. It was believed that while the patient was at home he would be closely monitored and his activities supervised by the same hospital staff of specialists. It was not the opinion of the patients and families that the family doctor would primarily manage the care. If he was to be involved at all, the family doctor was perceived as being a conduit between the patient and the specialist. This made immediate access to information somewhat less urgent since it was believed there would be ample opportunity later to get a thorough understanding of what had happened and its implications for the future lifestyle of the patient.

Most families were pleased that the patient had survived the heart attack and that he was going to be sent home eventually. They saw little reason to complain – even if they felt some amount of doubt and uncertainty about the details of the prognosis and future treatment regimen. In a couple of cases a false impression of the post hospital management was induced by residents who suggested that the hospital attending would follow up. Residents at Group Hospital can be unaware of the special procedures and systems used at Medical Group. They rotate through Group Hospital for three months, as part of their training. Prior to and afterward the residents train at the hospital which utilizes a more traditional system where family physicians are directly involved in the care of their hospitalized patients.

Being unfamiliar with the pre-paid group practice system can lead to problems. One event which I witnessed stands out from the rest. There was a patient on the ICU who was not given much chance of living if he did not have heart surgery. Yet, because of the patient's condition the surgery itself was considered to be a very risky procedure. As the time for a decision drew near, the resident who was involved with the patient said to a group, which included myself, gathered for coffee in the ICU foyer, that he was going to recommend to the family that the patient not have the operation because the chances were too slim and the cost of the operation would be very expensive to the family. At this moment, the head nurse was nearby and interrupted. "There is no cost to the family for the operation," she said, "they have paid a yearly premium for all care." The resident seemed surprised and taken aback that he had forgotten, and declared in that case he would recommend surgery. I heard him later that same day urge the patient, and the wife, to have the operation as the only chance of saving his life.

Another factor leading to the belief that the hospital based specialists would continue the care after hospitalization was the impression created among patients and family members alike that the family doctors were not trained to manage heart disease. There was little confusion, as I had initially expected there would be, over who would provide care for the patient in the hospital. The families seemed to accept easily the idea that specialists based in the hospital were the main providers of care here. They believed that heart attacks required experts specially trained in the care of the heart, and that the family physician who gave general care to family members for many "normal" health needs was just not trained to do this. Mrs Asti's comments on her family doctor are relevant here. I asked her what contact she had had with Dr C., her family physician: "Why would Dr C. want to see him, he's not a heart specialist. He's a different kind of doctor – he doesn't know about hearts. In fact, he had a heart attack himself once." Some patients like Mr Warren, were disappointed that the family doctor did not visit them in the hospital because it seemed to indicate a lack of concern. But no one complained that they would get better care by having the family doctor involved. On the contrary, patients and family members alike were agreed that the physician who treated their ills at the Medical Center was "only a general practitioner, and these guys [in the hospital] are specialists". Apart from being somewhat annoyed that the family doctor who sent them into the hospital never called or visited – just as patients were annoyed when certain friends or relatives didn't visit, it seemed quite logical that their general practitioners were not involved in the care. This extended to after hospital care.

When the time finally did come for the patient to leave the hospital, the promised discussion with the attending physician proved to be brief, with few concrete questions asked by patient or spouse. It would also prove to be largely inadequate for the needs of patients at home. In at least two cases, there would have been no discussion at all if a spouse had not accidentally come upon the physician on the day of discharge. Mrs Grasso was angry when she told me that only when she met the doctor by chance on the staircase as she was taking her husband out of the hospital did she receive instructions about the diet. The usual procedure was for the physician to give the patient a one day notice of hospital discharge. At that time he would tell the patient to prepare any questions he might have. In general the patients had few specific questions and their spouses had less.

The result was that many problems arose in the first few days following hospital discharge, which could have been anticipated and perhaps avoided with some prior thought. But the situation minimized the opportunity for the patient and his family to receive information, discuss it, and return with questions based on their thinking through the problem.

By the end of hospitalization it was apparent that the views of patients, family members, and medical staff were dissimilar. Trends that began to emerge early in the ICU continued for the duration of the hospital stay. Although during that time the setting and the care staff changed, the perceptual distance between the parties remained constant. In general, wives were less confident than their husbands that the illness which caused the hospitalization had been arrested, or that the need for hospitalization was over. The evidence indicates that neither medical staff nor nursing staff were conscious of the deep apprehension of the family members. At no time did the medical staff address itself to the indications of dissatisfaction and distrust manifested by the family members.

The patients seemed glad to be leaving the hospital, just as they had been relieved to be transferred to the General Medical Ward. However, this in no way indicated that the patients were emotionally prepared for the shift of care to the home, or that they adequately understood what they were to do once they got home. One need only recall the confusion and anxiety that attended the shift of patients from the ICU to the General Medical Ward.

There is no evidence at all that the hospital did not fulfill its responsibility to care for the patients' physical needs. In a space of a few weeks, patients who had arrived there in the most perilous straits were able to return to their families. This fact alone is a testimony to the efficiency and skill of the medical staff. Yet this improvement in health was accomplished with little participation of the patients themselves, or the members of their families. In effect, the patients were acted upon, and the organized routines of the care setting served to prevent them from interfering with the goals of the institution.

If the illness were of the acute type such an approach might be sufficient. However, the patients did not leave the hospital cured of their medical problem. Hospital discharge merely marked the end of one phase of treatment and the beginning of another. The setting of care and rehabilitation would now be the home where the attitudes and understanding of all the family members would take on a new importance. It is this reality that was not taken into account by the efficient, bureaucratically-oriented care system of Group Hospital.

Transferring Responsibility from Hospital to Home

The passage of the patient from the hospital ward to the familiar surroundings of home might be expected to be a time of relief and celebration in the family. Davis (1963:83) reported that when the day of homecoming finally arrived for the families he studied, "A reunion glow suffused the life of the family; doubts were temporarily laid aside, and a determined effort was made to 'look on the bright side of things'." This was not the case for the families I studied. Upon the arrival of the heart patient home from the hospital, the atmosphere in each of the eight families was suffused with worried concern. The patient's removal from direct medical supervision seemed to cause the family members a high degree of apprehension over whether he could be safe with only his family to look after him.

The day of homecoming set the tone for the days, and in the case of some families the weeks, that were to follow. There were no celebrations or ritual events to mark the passage from hospital to home, or to give any indication that a new status for the husband–patient had been achieved. By everyone's account the men appeared reluctant to explore the home they had been absent from for several weeks, and their families urged them to spend the day in bed, or at least to sit reading or watching television. Not only were there no celebrations, but there was also a deliberate attempt to transform the home into a quiet, restful place for the sick. This pattern was the same in all families but one. Against his wife's strenuous objections, Mr Polski insisted on accompanying her to the store where he waited in the car while she shopped. However, he later admitted that he should not have gone since he became very tired. For the rest of the day, and for the next several days, his behavior was very much like that of the other men: he remained almost exclusively in bed or in a chair.

On the basis of what I was told by family members, and what I personally observed in the first two weeks following hospital discharge, it seems reasonable to characterize this period as the *Period of Extension of Hospitalization.* In response to the anxiety generated by the homecoming, particularly around the issue of preventing any circumstances from arising that would cause the men to be placed under physical or mental stress, wives, children, and the patient–husbands themselves tried to incorporate into the home atmosphere the safeguards they had witnessed (and felt secure in) in the hospital, especially those of the Intensive Care Unit. This included the men assuming the patient role typical of acute illness, with wives and children acting the part of nurse–surrogates. These roles emphasized passivity and inactivity for the husband and close surveillance by his wife and children. One of the major characteristic features of the *Period of Extension of Hospitalization* was that the men at home were all less active than they had been in their final days in the hospital. In terms of willingness to test themselves by walking or lifting small objects, which most men had done in the hospital, their present reluctance to do much more than sit or sleep represents a regression to earlier stage of illness.

Each of the wives I spoke with about this period believed that she had an important but difficult responsibility: making the home environment as safe as possible for the husband–patient. Practically speaking, this included preventing any but the most necessary activity on the man's part, discouraging visitors, keeping strict control over food preparation, and protecting him from situations that might cause any anxiety. Wives were particularly careful that household chores were taken care of so he "won't worry about it." One of the sources of the wife's sense of obligation for the husband–patient's safety, and consequently of her willingness to work so hard, was the fear that his health was so fragile that it was subject to sudden renewed reinjury with little provocation. Moreover, the family had observed in the hospital that the patient tended to do too much, according to its perception of his care needs. Wives and children believed that their role was to continue the function of protecting the patient from the environment, and, very importantly, from his own acts.

Wives and children watched the husband–patients just as they had been constantly monitored and observed in the ICU, and they tried to keep them immobile. One husband said: "If I drop a piece of paper, she won't let me pick it up." I asked another: "Are you both in agreement on the amount of activity you should be getting?" He answered: "Oh yeah. She is right on my tail – don't, don't do it." Just as the ICU nurses told them not to do anything without being assisted and to let the nurses take care of their needs, the wives also expected their husbands to rely on them. Mrs Warren said: "If he wants to help me lift anything, I'll say 'No, I'll do it.' He has not gone down the steps to check the water in the boiler yet: I won't let him."

When a man even accidently attempted anything considered potentially dangerous by the wife, he was checked by a sharp word from her. She used the same means to control patient behavior as the ICU nurse had – by reminding him of his susceptibility to reinjury, and demanding compliance.

The fears of the wives at this time were dramatically conveyed in stories I was told by a number of them, relating incidents in which relatives or neighbors had died of heart attacks suddenly, even "right outside of the doctors office," or, "just as he came home from the doctor." These fears were probably behind the lengths to which wives went in order to monitor and supervise the men's activities. Those women who had jobs stayed home, at least for the first several days. All altered their normal schedules to be in the home, even in the same room as the sick person.

These stories of sudden death were in many respects like the ones told to me by the ICU nurses of patients who died on the ward following exertion. The similarity suggests that nurses responsible for new heart patients, and wives in their role of nurse–surrogate who feel responsible for newly discharged heart patients, share a common set of problems. Both are cognizant of the limitations of medical science to cure the illness. The stories told by nurses and wives all stress that patients died in or near a medical setting, and with little forewarning. Both nurse and wife worried that even the well-intentioned patient was capable of dangerous overactivity, and both felt accountable for preventing situations from arising that might threaten the patient's chances for survival. By "doing everything possible" to counteract any attempt by the patient to be autonomous or active, the care givers shield themselves from the possibility of guilt or blame in the event of death. The enforcement of extensive limitations of activity may be seen as a way of adapting to the high degree of uncertainty in the situation. The ritualistic application of a set of controls, which in its rigidity went beyond what was required by medical guidelines, may also be conceived of as a functional equivalent of magic. As Parsons (1951:469) explains, "The basic function of magic . . . is to bolster the self confidence of actors in situations where energy and skill *do* make a difference but where because of uncertainty factors, outcomes cannot be guaranteed." The wives believed they would have much to do with quality of the husband–patient's health once they left the hospital. They were highly involved emotionally. Yet, they were uncertain whether the goals to which they were committed were achievable in the home setting. Their actions seemed to be an attempt to re-create the safe atmosphere of the ICU. By following precisely what they had seen done by ICU nurses, the wives hoped to stand between the men and disaster. Not only was it hoped that this highly restrictive approach would offer more certainty that the patient would suffer no harm, but it reduced the amount of individual judgement required.

Another characteristic of the *Period of Extension of Hospitalization* was the absence of interpersonal conflict in the families. Couples who regularly argued before the illness seemed to be in accord during this period. When a wife became upset because the man did not want to take another nap, or when she noticed him doing something like putting a dinner plate into the sink, it seemed like a word from her was usually sufficient to cause him to comply with what he was told. Children also were more likely to offer to help their mother, and in the case of the Asti children there was a moratorium on arguing. Rose Asti said she could not remember a time when she and her brother John got along so well.

At this point one could argue that the family members

perceived the crisis as having been imposed on the family by forces outside the control of anyone in the group. No one, therefore, could be blamed for the troubles the family was having. Responding to an external threat seemed to heighten the members sense of loyalty to one another and, consequently, affective interpersonal relations strengthened the integrity of the family bond.

In contrast to the harmony between individuals, they shared an acute sense of fear and doubt about the illness reoccurring. This was reinforced whenever the man felt even slight discomfort.

From the comments made by family members during this time, it is apparent that a small amount of chest pain which might be expected to arise occasionally in the recovering heart patient, and for which several patients had received medication (nitroglycerine), was enough to reaffirm the family resolve to prevent any unnecessary patient activity. Not only chest pain, but any sign that the patient-husband was unwell was cause for continuing alarm. Mrs Asti was concerned because her husband's feet were cold at night. She said they never were before. To her, this was indicative of the man's fragile state of health.

Mr and Mrs Goldberg's reaction was not untypical. My statement, "I guess it's nice to have your husband home," led Mrs Goldberg to make the following comments:

> Yes, but it's very worrisome. It's very uncertain. I'm very frightened, let me put it that way . . . Last night he said he wasn't feeling that good, and it's very upsetting. You wonder: What's going to happen now . . . I told him: "Why fight it. Go to bed" . . . I didn't know how bad he felt. He said this morning, "Gee, I didn't think I'd make it." I don't know if he was exaggerating or whether he was scared. He [said he had] a slight pain up here. It's not all healed.

On another occasion, a complaint of a slight pain made Mrs Goldberg feel ill herself. Another wife, Mrs Ambrosio said that when she held her husband in bed she could feel that "his heart was irregular" and she wept.

For Mr O'Shea the days following hospital discharge were "worse than when I went into the hospital." He said he felt "run down, and washed out." When I asked why he didn't feel "washed out" in the hospital he replied then that "something's going on all the time. I wasn't by myself thinking, thinking." One of the things he was thinking about was whether he was doing what his doctor advised. Before he left the hospital he was told "not to tire myself." He was also told to nap during the day. However, Mr O'Shea found himself unable to nap – "my mind keeps active" – and by nightfall he would feel fatigued. This led him to worry about whether he was getting worse, which was on his mind when he tried to nap. To compensate for his inability to nap he tried to remain sedentary and when I asked him to compare the amount of activity, including walking, he had now with what he had in the hospital, he replied that he did more in the hospital.

The recovering men, and their families displayed a high need for reassurance that healing was taking place. They were impatient for the first visit with a doctor, particularly a heart specialist. In a subsequent chapter I will take up the issue of the family's concern that the family physician was not qualified to handle the heart patient's needs. For now I merely want to point out that the time between hospital discharge and the first doctor's visit was experienced by the family in such a way as to heighten the anxiety and to increase their dependency on the health care system.

Waiting to be seen by the doctor was, as Mrs Goldberg put it "like waiting for the Lord." I happened to be present when Mr Ambrosio received in the mail his appointment slip for the first post-hospital electrocardiogram. His reaction was a combination of relief and jubilation.

At the outset of home care, patients and family members waited anxiously for the medical care system to resume direct control over patient management. Given the doubts and fears they labored under, two or three weeks appeared to the family members as a terribly long time to have to wait to learn if the man had improved or gotten worse. For some people it seemed as if they had been abandoned. Mr Ambrosio expressed this sentiment to me in the following way.

I think it is a glaring fault of the system. I'm home now roughly ten days and no one has called from the hospital;

neither social service or medical to see how I'm feeling. . . .
While you are in there [the hospital] you get all this positive
approach. Everyone is trying to help you: Do this, do that,
get your food, get rest and all that. Then when you get
home. . . .

Mr O'Shea called the hospital for help in getting a
prescription filled. He was discharged from the hospital on
New Year's day and could not find a drug store open. The
following day his family was in a state of panic, because the
local pharmacist told them he thought this particular drug
had been discontinued. Mr O'Shea recalled these events:

I was without [the medication] over a day already. I was
starting to sweat it out and finally I says "let me get in touch
with the hospital and see what goes on." I asked for Dr A
. . . I says to him: "How's the chance of getting [the
medication] in the pharmacy there?" He said, "I don't
think they fill prescriptions there for people not in the
hospital." Finally, that day about 5.30 pm, the druggist
found it and sent it over. That was quite a relief . . . It
shook me up something terrible. I don't think I recovered
from that yet.

A problem which several families faced during the early
days of the home care was how to manage the diet. At least
three families believed they were supposed to follow a diet
regimen but were given no written instructions. Mrs Goldberg said she was told, "since he's an old diabetic just feed
him like before." However she told me, "we've gotten away
from his diet for a long time now so I really don't know what
to feed him." Mrs Asti thought her husband was told to
follow a low caloric diet. She did not know what this meant.
Since the first appointment with the doctor was two weeks
away she tried to remember what her husband had been fed in
the hospital. Her uncertainty over the adequacy of the food
she was preparing caused her considerable upset. She was
very impatient for the opportunity to discuss this with the
doctor. The Warren's did receive written instructions concerning the diet regimen on the day Mr Warren left the
hospital. However, during my first visit with the family

shortly after homecoming, both spouses reported that it was complex and ambiguous. They hoped that I could help them clarify what the instructions meant precisely, because they felt at a loss to do so themselves. Doubts about the diet again made the hospital care the model to follow at home. Until they could see the doctor, they would be as cautious as possible, and the members searched their memories for what they had seen while in the hospital.

The start of the home care phase of recovery from heart attack seems to contain a number of elements that operate to *increase* the patient's and the family's *dependency* on the health care system. Consequently, progress toward rehabilitation comes to a halt and even regresses for a period following hospital discharge. Without the presence of medical experts to direct and reassure him, the heart patient at home can become immobilized. Moreover, while the family members were actively involved in patient care at home, their actions were directed toward maintaining a hospital-like atmosphere, resulting in a parody of the ICU. Every attempt was made *not* to develop autonomous rehabilitation roles, but to enforce a pattern of behavior appropriate for patients in an acute state of illness.

The reaction following hospital discharge parallels that which some men experienced when they were transferred from the ICU to the general medical ward. Then, the reduction of direct professional supervision also caused several men to seek security in highly sedentary behavior. Recall also that the transfer heightened the worry of the family members with the result that many of them tried to compensate by protecting the men from activity. At each point, when the setting of care seemed to provide the opportunity for greater patient-family autonomy, the result was *more not less*, dependence on restrictions, and commitment to the passive–dependent sick role. At least at the outset of home care, all patients and wives and children were fearful of dread consequences of the illness. For a short time, all the patients acted like "cardiac cripples" in that their fear of reinjury prevented them from behaving up to their potential.

According to the observations made of eight families, one is able to note that unless the patient and his family are ready to assume the responsibility for care, there is the danger that the withdrawal of medical support will be perceived by them as threatening to the patient's well being, and will cause the family to try to compensate for it by adopting a highly conservative stance toward treatment, a negative outlook for the future, and an inflated view of their need for continuous medical attention. One cannot help but note, however, that such consequences as these seem inevitable given the suddenness with which the transition from hospital to home took place.

When the care system discharged the patient from the hospital, it left the family on its own. Preparing the family for home care with a few general guidelines and advising that a physicians appointment be made in two or three weeks, the care system left the patient and his spouse to grapple with the day-to-day complexities of the care alone. It provided no mechanisms for linking the family with the care system, at least until the first visit to the physician. Decisions with regard to helping the patient, or adjustments to slight but worrisome changes in the way the patient was feeling were placed entirely on the family. The care system acted as if the patient and family were able to be self-reliant without any preparation. As a consequence, there was no way of knowing whether the actions that the family was taking at home were consistent with the expectations of the medical care system.

4

Family Lifestyles

So far in our analysis of the situation that the families were facing we have given a central place to the hospital and its social organization with reference to the procedures and arrangements for managing the patients' care. This includes ways of handling family members during hospitalization. It was necessary to look closely at these institutional factors because they provided the major point of reference for the families in their understanding of the immediate problem and with dealing with it on an emotional level. We also wanted to point out some of the unintended and latent short- and long-range consequences of the way medical care for heart patients is organized.

At this point, however, we must turn our attention to the families' inner lives and look closely at the major components of their affective and instrumental relationships. The families, at this stage of recovery, would be faced with decisions about incorporating the therapeutic plan, as this was understood by the various members, into a stream of everyday activities which are necessary for maintaining a functioning unit. Some balance had to be reached between normal life activities and the new requirements. The patients' needs would now be viewed against those of others in the family. This is the nature of coping.

In their article, "A Framework for Studying Families in Crisis," Parad and Caplan (1965:57) addressed the point I have just made in the following terms. They stated that, "When the family faces a stressful event, its life style places at its disposal a range of problem-solving possibilities from which the family members individually and collectively may choose according to their perceptions of the demands of the

83

situation." By "life style" they refer to the family's value system, communication network, and role system. In other words, families who face similar problems develop strategies for coping with them in ways that are compatible with what Handel (1972) refers to as the psychosocial interior of the family. Parad and Caplan go on to explain that,

> the essence of a crisis is that the situation cannot be easily handled by the family's commonly used problem-solving mechanisms, but forces the employment of novel patterns. These are necessarily within the range of the family's capacities, but may be patterns never called into operation in the past.

Insofar as these eight families were in a stage of their life cycles where changing patterns of living are likely to occur, the present crisis was not dissimilar in some of its effects to what was occurring naturally. Retirement had brought about role changes in some cases and the anticipation of retirement and relocation had initiated anticipation of changes in living patterns in other families. Serious illness had occurred, as well as other traumatic events, such as a child's divorce. So adjusting to yet another serious challenge was not an entirely novel situation. Yet the essence of Parad and Caplan's insight is that, while coping with crisis may be within the family's capacity, the outcome may depend upon the present life situation of individual members, which colors their perceptions of the events that are taking place. Particularly in groups where change is already occurring, *negotiated* problem solving is essential.

In this chapter, the essential features of the families' interior lives will be sketched. Included will be the major concerns that were occupying their everyday lives at the time the attack struck.

The data on family life obtained through the interviews with family members will be discussed around two related concepts: the first is the family's pattern of separateness and connectedness. I am using Hess and Handel's (1959:5) notion that, "the family tries to cast itself in a form that satisfies the ways in which its members want to be together and apart." Within the extremes of isolated separateness and stifling connectedness, there is a wide range of ways in which family members may achieve a balance between being separate and together. We in no way want to place a value judgment on which works best. Members who exercise considerable independence over their activities and spend large blocks of time engaged in separate endeavors outside the home may feel the bond between themselves and their families as intensely or more so than those whose activities are more constrained by familial requirements.

We looked at the family division of labor to ascertain the mechanisms by which essential functions of the group were carried out. Were roles highly differentiated with clear normative boundaries surrounding each, or were roles defined more on a sharing and exchanging of functions?

While analytically distinct, the two concepts seem, in reality, to be linked. For example, the need to feel connected with others may give rise to a highly differentiated role structure in which the performance of most functions requires reciprocity and concordance of individual activities. In families of this type, which included two among our eight, the Grassos and the Goldbergs, members are dependent upon others in the family to provide a range of day-to-day services, and since roles are not normally interchangeable, failure of one person to fulfill his or her obligations deprives the others of services they come to expect. In these families the members, particularly the spouses, find their emotional gratification within the boundaries of the nuclear unit. Connectedness is manifested by reciprocity within the home and joint participation in social spheres outside of the home.

In four of our families – the Astis, Polskis, Steins, and Warrens – flexibility with regard to when and by whom tasks were accomplished was expected. Each person performed a range of family tasks and did not depend nearly as much on the role performances of others. These were families in which the members derived considerable satisfaction in activities they engaged in separately, in and outside of the home. A highly differentiated structure would have imposed constraints on the flexibility required to meet individuals' personal interests and social obligations. These families appeared similar to some of the "dual-career" families studied by the Rapaports (1971:108), in which, "The emphasis is placed on different activities as demands change – [where there is] a lack of emphasis on 'servicing' one another, but rather an emphasis on individuals looking after themselves." These were not people who were isolated or who felt estranged from the family, rather they valued their membership precisely because of the social space it provided them.

Rounding out our group of families, there were two – the Ambrosios and the O'Sheas – in which a satisfactory balance of separateness and connectedness had not been achieved. With the O'Sheas, the issue revolved around physical presence and companionship. Mrs O'Shea argued that her husband was too involved in outside activities with church and community affairs to provide her with the companionship she felt entitled to. Her sense of connectedness required her husband's physical presence. With the Ambrosios, the issue was over roles. She exhibited what may be described as role deprivation due to her husband's insistence on assuming, since his retirement from full-time employment, the largest share of household tasks, including those she felt were within a wife's domain. Both husbands insisted on their right to choose themselves when and how they participated in the home.

Researchers often attempt to deal with the complexity of modern marriage and family life through categories that are both analytically relevant and descriptive of some major interactive element. For example, Hicks and Platt (1970), in a review of research on marital stability, assert that, at least two basic marital types co-exist in the United States: the institutional and the companionship. Pratt (1976) has described a type of family which fosters a healthy lifestyle in its members as "energized." Families have at different times been described as egalitarian, traditional, atomized, and so on. Each of these is a way of capturing the essence of marital and family relations as it relates to the issues that are being addressed. We have found the terms *convergence* and *divergence* to reflect interactional patterns that appear most salient to the issue of coping with heart disease.

The terms convergence and divergence are meant to suggest the fundamental orientation of family values and role arrangements. Convergence suggests a focus inward, with primacy given to what members of a group may do together rather than separately. In contrast, divergence implies an outward focus, with primacy given to members' individualized needs and priorities.

Divergence in Family Life – The Astis, Polskis, Steins, and Warrens

Each of the divergent families in some important way manifested the value of separateness over connectedness. Members of these four households placed a significant amount of emphasis on activities engaged in alone. Family routines accommodated members' independent pursuits and, at the same time, provided enough of a group focus so that members had regular and, according to them, satisfying family relationships. What distinguishes these families is the emphasis on social and emotional resources apart from those derived from within the nuclear unit.

Mr and Mrs Stein spend a good deal of time apart because of their different work schedules. He works at his job as a photoengraver during the evening hours, and she as a secretary during the day. The couple interacts face-to-face only on weekends. During the week, they communicate with one another by phone and through written messages. Time spent together was, however, described as warm and congenial, and they actually attribute the success of their relationship to the fact that "there is no time for fighting." Neither considers the opportunity to spend more time together as a sufficient reason for seeking a change in either person's employment.

Both Mr and Mrs Stein value their privacy. Once home, she not infrequently would disconnect the telephone in order not to be interrupted as she watched TV or took care of household chores. Mr Stein spent long hours after work planning his investments. This activity, which he considered a hobby and which entertained and relaxed him, was not shared by his wife. In fact, she claimed to take no interest in these investments, leaving the matter of how much to invest entirely to her husband. On weekends the couple caught up on accumulated chores. Their approach to this was casual since neither enjoyed very much house cleaning, gardening, repairing, or planning and shopping for meals, and other similar activities. There was some pattern to their activities in the home. Mrs Stein more often cleaned the home, and Mr Stein usually expected to keep the garden neat and take care of large home repairs. But even here there was overlap, because each tended to minimize the amount of time spent in these activities. Mrs Stein, for example, saw to the gardening if she felt it was being neglected. Her husband straightened up the house when it became too sloppy for his taste. Neither expressed criticism of the way the other carried out these functions. In addition to doing most of his own cooking, Mr Stein also helped his wife plan for the shopping by specifying what foods he would like purchased. She usually purchased the food. As far as serving meals, this chore was shared. They ate their meals on weekends while watching television, and depending on who was more involved in the program, or who was more tired, one or the other served the meal.

The Polskis maintain two households, one in the city, in the neighborhood where Mrs Polski grew up and has a number of close friends and ties to the local church; the other in a suburb fifty miles away which Mr Polski built himself. The couple have had problems deciding how much time to spend in each of their homes. In recent years they have dealt with this by living apart for periods of time, from days to weeks, on a regular basis. As mentioned, Mrs Polski derives a great deal of pleasure being in the company of her friends in the city. Mr Polski enjoys boating with his friends in the suburbs and also has numerous projects around the larger suburban home and property. He does not socialize with his wife and her friends when in the city. This arrangement, while not without its limitations, allows each spouse the opportunity to engage in valued social pursuits. Although each would like to spend even more time in their respective preferred domiciles, the present pattern seems to have reduced past tensions to an acceptable level.

The pace of life in the Warren household was quite slow. Since retirement, the couple has not found much to do with their time. Mr Warren spends many hours each day watching television while Mrs Warren "usually just mopes around," doing crossword puzzles, sewing, and sitting in the garden. Even though in close proximity, the couple attested to the fact that they did few things together or even held much conversation during the course of a normal day. This seemed to reflect their general passivity and not hostility toward one another. They were members of a local church and did attend social functions together.

Taking care of household chores seemed to provide a relief from the day's routine. Such activities as shopping or taking the laundry to be cleaned were attended to by one of the spouses according to who seemed inclined. In all, the content of the day's activities depended on personal inclination rather than any organized plan.

Both Mr and Mrs Asti take considerable pride in home ownership and work hard at keeping the house and grounds in good repair. Mr Asti was content to spend his spare time doing household chores. However, he insisted on controlling what he did and when he did it. When asked for occasions of conflict with his wife, he identified times when she has tried to tell him what chores to do when he had other plans. When asked what qualities he most admired in his wife, he responded: "Like me, she never calls a tradesman to do repairs but does them herself." She even had her own toolbox for making household repairs. While it was Mr Asti's habit to do major repairs around the house, and to service the family cars, he was not pleased with this arrangement, and had been trying to involve his wife and daughter more in these activities. For example, he wanted them to know how to make minor repairs on the cars and to keep them serviced. He claimed that since they drive, this is useful information, and being dependent on him limited their own ability to be self-reliant, a quality he admires in people.

The family commitment to individual choice was evident when occasions arose when Mr Asti would ask one of the children for help with some chore around the house. It was understood that their son's and daughter's priorities came first, and there was no insistence that a child help at home when he or she had something else planned. No pressure or threat of reprisal accompanied a refusal of one member of the family to help another. The parents were actually hesitant to seek the assistance of their children partly because they may have had to wait for the children to become free to help. Parents had definite ideas about how they wanted chores done and preferred doing them themselves, thus guaranteeing a certain level of task performance. Mr Asti said: "John has a tendency to forget – like taking out the garbage. That's why I try to do a lot of things myself." Notice that there is no attempt to insist that John conform to his father's expectations.

The children were not in the habit of informing their parents when they would be out, or when they could come home. There was no constraint on them to take meals at home. If someone missed a meal, he or she cooked separately. Mrs Asti would leave the food on the stove for anyone to reheat. Although Mrs Asti regularly cooked dinner, she exerted no control over the behavior of others around meals. Her role as family cook was not one that called forth a reciprocal response from others, and stands as an example of the general lack of interdependence of members in the household.

The spouses pursued independent recreational activities. Mrs Asti had her own set of friends whom she saw weekday afternoons and weekend evenings. There was some joint recreating – both spouses like to go to play bingo at the local church – but each enjoyed leisure activities the other did not. The result was that each found companions with whom these interests could be expressed.

I asked the members to describe the way conflicts were most often resolved in the home. Mrs Asti said: "We try to ignore one another." Rose said that when one of her parents is in a "nasty mood" she spends more time away from home until the atmosphere has changed.

To summarize, while these families are unique in many respects, they share an approach to living together. I have chosen to label this approach divergence. It is manifested in the way everyday life is organized, which is around the exchange of roles so that members are not dependent upon one another for services. Reciprocity is limited to the granting of social space for individual pursuits. Problem solving within the nuclear unit involves increasing social distance in order to accomodate individual differences. In a real sense, members are not dependent upon the family for self-actualization.

Convergence in Family Life: Grassos and Goldbergs

In the two families I have labeled convergent, the pattern is different: individuals' interests yield to those of the group. Interdependence is fostered by a role-differentiated family structure and a strong value placed on face-to-face interaction and joint participation with social networks. Problem solving, moreover, involves give and take until a solution is arrived at which is consistent with the values of the group. In a real sense, the nuclear unit is the focus of individual fulfilment.

In the Grasso family, a persistent source of friction between husband and wife involves the amount of time Mr Grasso spends on his work. As the manager of the family business, a small grocery store, he often feels he must work long hours. Following his first heart attack, the idea of a small business was conceived as an alternative to other types of employment which were thought to be more physically and emotionally demanding. Mrs Grasso feels that since she works full time, financial need does not necessitate her husband's aggressive approach to his work. His absence from the home, she feels, deprives her of his companionship, and since she will not visit relatives and friends alone, or engage in any other out-of-the-home recreation by herself, Mr Grasso's behavior limits both her mobility and her leisure. For his part, Mr Grasso accepts his wife's criticism as valid. He readily agrees that his wife had a right to expect his companionship and expressed sympathy for the deprivation she felt. However, he claimed that the business was just beginning to show profits and he did not want to see his efforts to build the business go for naught. Moreover, owning and operating a successful business was consistent with the image of masculinity he desired to have and project. He admitted he would deeply regret having to depend on his wife's income. He seemed to feel caught between his need to insure a positive self-image based on his occupational role and economic leadership in the family and his felt obligations to his wife.

Parent–child relationships in the Grasso family provide a sharp contrast with those described above in the Asti family. Anthony, twenty-two years old, was formerly married and has a child, and at the time of his father's heart attack was managing a restaurant and living at home. Yet in the home, both he and his parents emphasized that he was still subject to parental restrictions. For example, if he was not going to be home by a certain time in the evening, he was required to call his parents and let them know when to expect him. Mr and Mrs Grasso felt that they still had an obligation to guide and counsel their son. Mrs Grasso was disappointed that Anthony left college for his present position and had been making an extensive effort to persuade him to return. In the home there was regular sharing of interests. Father and son watched and discussed sports, and they attended sporting events together. At the dinner table, politics and religion were discussed, with the father and son usually disagreeing with Mrs Grasso.

In the Grasso and Goldberg families, the practice of having family tasks allocated along traditional lines of sex and generation was valued by all the members. In both families, the wives were responsible for traditional female tasks of shopping for and preparing food, all regular house cleaning, mending and laundering clothing, decorating the home, etc. The husbands had some housekeeping chores – cleaning walls, moving furniture, making structural repairs, caring for the family car, and other male-oriented tasks, including their role as economic provider.

Mrs Grasso worked four days a week. She began when her children were in their teens. She and her husband reported that it was agreed beforehand that she would continue to do all the household chores and would leave her job if it interfered with the smooth functioning of the household.

On any given evening during the week, the observer in the home might witness Mrs Grasso doing the following chores until after 11 pm: cooking, dishes, laundry or ironing, light housekeeping, preparing her clothing and person for the next day's work. During this time, her husband and son might be watching TV. There was no expectation that either should assist her in these chores although they often kept her company by talking with her when she worked. After dinner Mr Grasso recorded the day's receipts from the family business. He put stock for the next day into his car – it was stored in the basement – and then was free to do his own household chores, or watch TV, read, and do whatever he pleased. The family's friends followed the same pattern, I was told. On the other hand, Mrs Grasso had no hand in the operation of the family business, which was her husband's responsibility.

Yet the role-differentiated style of living brought the couples together on a regular basis. For example, the activity of food buying, preparation, and serving was the sole responsibility of the wives in the Grasso and Goldberg families. But transportation was the husbands' task. Both sets of spouses went to the market together, but the husbands had little or no input into what was purchased. Mealtimes in the role-differentiated families were joint activities. Members were expected to eat together. If someone wanted to be absent, he was required to notify the woman in advance. Since she had the responsibility of preparing meals, the wife expected others to respond by being present. She had control over these aspects of the family's activities.

Discordance in Family Life: Ambrosios and O'Sheas

The relationship between family organization and individual need-gratification comes into sharp focus when examining daily life in the two discordant families. Both wives were very often unsuccessful at having their husbands adhere to a segregated system of task responsibilities, which would have brought husband and wife together on a more regular basis.

The Ambrosios are a retired couple with two married children. In telling me of their childrearing days, Mrs Ambrosio spoke of the pleasure she took from her homemaking role. She recalled:

I have friends when their husbands are coming in the door from work they don't know what they are going to make. I think a table should be set when a man comes home from

work. That is part of a home. When I observe that I say I'm
never going to complain. That is a joy, to have the food
ready. They say, "What am I going to take from the
freezer?" I always plan the day before; and then look
forward to making it. When the kids would come home
from school, they would say, "What have you got?" They
would take the cover off, open the oven. We used to do that
at home.

Before her husband retired, she was "in control of"
housekeeping chores like shopping and preparing food,
housecleaning, and bill paying. As noted above, she enjoyed
being responsible for and carrying out this function.

Studies show that after retirement it is not unusual for a
man to participate in some aspects of tasks formerly done
exclusively by the wife. But as Ballweg (1967) points out, the
assumption by the husband of additional household duties
need not constitute a disturbing force in the relationship. In
the Ambrosio family, however, it did. Since his retirement,
Mr Ambrosio has attempted to assume the major functionary
role in the home. By his remarkable energy – he said he has
slept no more than four hours a night all of his adult life – he
has been able to initiate chores before his wife has a chance to
do them. The following is part of his description of his typical
morning prior to his heart attack:

My normal procedure is to get up early, make the coffee,
have a cup, get the newspapers, pick up the milk from my
friend who has a fruit stand, be back by 7–7.30, have
another cup of coffee, read the paper, and by 8.00 I am in
the supermarket. (Observer E.S. "When is your wife up?")
I told her to sleep. She sleeps. When I get up she says,
"Where are you going?" I say, "Go back to bed. I'm going
to get up." "What can you do, it is still dark." By nine I
have avoided the rush at the supermarket, got all the
goodies done.

Having these household duties taken from her has had a
profound effect on Mrs Ambrosio. In commenting on her
feelings about this she revealed a negative self-image as a
result of having a minimal family role: "I feel so stupid in so

many things. For instance like the light doesn't go on. He always does it, does everything . . . and I don't know how. I feel like now he should let me."

During the interviews, she spoke of her husband's failure to acknowledge her ability to accomplish meaningful tasks around the house, thereby making her feel like a child. What she would like is to be identified with a wider range of activities similar to those she had prior to her husband's retirement and have her husband respect her hegemony over these areas of their joint life. He then would be her role partner. She would like her husband to remain responsible for "the masculine chores," painting, repairing, taking out the garbage, etc., but not chores in her domain: preparing meals, shopping for food, cleaning, etc.

In the retirement phase Mrs Ambrosio often has tried to recapture some of the prized household activities for herself. Over her husband's objections she would meet him at the train station with the car in inclement weather, buy him clothes, and generally try to establish some control of family functions. She has regularly attempted to influence what is purchased at the supermarket. Sometimes this contest results in task duplication. For example, after Mr Ambrosio has cleaned the kitchen his wife will repeat this chore when he has finished. She has often insisted that it is her job to do this.

Mrs Ambrosio was a member of a number of community organizations in which she has risen to a position of leadership. She told me that she joined them because she had nothing to do at home and would gladly end her participation if the pattern at home were altered.

In spite of her extensive out-of-the-home role, her most significant point of reference is her husband and her family, and her vision of an ideal family situation includes husband and wife linked through the coordination of separate activities, dependent upon each other, respectful of each other's domain, sharing some activities, including decision making, and being regular companions to each other. Without his cooperation, she cannot actualize her life goals.

There is a similar issue active in the *O'Shea family*. Mrs O'Shea, like Mrs Ambrosio, values high role differentiation and what this implies for reciprocal, coordinated behavior.

Mrs O'Shea perceives the marital relationships as comprising an array of reciprocal role relationships bearing on various aspects of marriage and family life. Mr O'Shea's conception is more narrowly drawn. An example of their general contention is over housekeeping roles. Mr O'Shea would like dinner, for example, to be an activity which members participate in according to their outside priorities. If he is late from work, or has a community meeting to attend, he prefers to make his own dinner when it is convenient for him. But in his wife's view, preparing dinner is an activity covered by her role as wife, and his absence deprives the role of meaning. Outside activities should not interfere. It is a meaningful part of her role if he reciprocates the activity and partakes of the meal at the time it is prepared. She perceives her various housekeeping roles as containing privileges as well as obligations, including the right to organize the participation of others. She wants to mark clearly the distinctions in the family over tasks and stresses the needed complementary of their roles. Some specific areas of contention in the family are: transportation – she wants to shop, but wants him to drive her; housecleaning – she wants to define which chores will regularly be performed by what person.

An important issue for Mrs O'Shea is companionship. Because of his extensive community involvement, Mr O'Shea is out of the house most evenings. His wife is home alone. She argues that as her husband, he is obliged to give her companionship. He argues that she should not rely only on him, but find substitute companions. Although she has friends with whom she socializes, her notion is that her status as wife is limited by her husband's unwillingness to act as a suitable role partner and companion.

Both of these wives are selective in their preferred view of how family relationships should be ordered. Like Mrs Ambrosio, there are some family activities Mrs O'Shea definitely does not want her husband to be involved with. Her selection is also along traditional male–female lines. She does not want him to do laundry, or cook, or take an active role in decorating the house.

In the chapters that follow, we shall explore the relevance of these family and conjugal patterns for coping with the demands of recovery from heart attack. We shall see that the desire in the recovery process to remain compatible with highly valued personal and family goals can conflict with definitions of the situation held by medical professionals involved in the patient's care or with obligations members themselves feel they have in representing the medical system's perspective in the home. The tensions engendered by such a conflict can become an important source of personal and group discontent. However, such a set of circumstances may also lead members to redefine the situation by reformulating rehabilitation priorities and reinterpreting the health needs of the member–patient. It is reasonable to expect that people will generally try to minimize the threat to their psychological and social well-being and maximize opportunities for stable, fulfilling relationships. We will explore the hypothesis that the way the recovery process is perceived and organized in families reflects the desire either to stabilize family relationships which show signs of deteriorating under the stress of illness or to bring about changes in basic family patterns which some members feel are needed to correct an imablance between family goals and family routines which pre-existed the illness onset.

5

Coping at Home:
Problems and Adjustments

In the early home care period it was pointed out that there was little tendency for the family members to engage together in discussions of patient activity. Questions of what the patient could and could not do rarely came up. At home, the patient simply did as little as possible. As Mr Ambrosio put it, "When in doubt, do nothing." Everyone subscribed to this orientation.

Agreement over the means of coping with the management of the recovery process, which characterized the early days of home care, began to break down as soon as the husband–patients made their first tentative moves toward activity.

At first, the men undertook simple activities like cleaning the dinner dishes, or setting the dinner table, changing light bulbs, and the like, and when they discovered they could accomplish these activities without discomfort, they attempted slightly more substantial tasks, for example, carrying a bag of garbage from the kitchen to a pail in the pantry. It is important to note that these were done without prior consultation with either physician or spouse. The men, it seemed, were attempting quietly to test their stamina against what they thought were fairly safe activities.

Usually the first significant task attempted involved something that was clearly identified with their normal role at home and that others, even in divergent families, did not normally share. Two men went down to the basement to check the heating system. One of them, Mr Stein, told me that even though he realized that his wife had been handling this chore successfully in his absence, he felt he had to check it for himself. "I must see that you are doing it right," he said to his wife when she objected to his going down the stairs. Mr Ambrosio felt he had to check on a small crack in his basement wall to determine if it needed repair. With this goal in mind he went down a flight of steps for the first time in spite of his wife's objections.

At this time, these recently discharged patients took steps to be less visible to their spouses, who were becoming increasingly concerned over the subtle but certain turn of events. Earlier, the men tended to stay in places where they could easily be observed – the kitchen or the living room. All social establishments, Goffman tells us, have norms that govern what behavior is acceptable in the various spatial settings that comprise it. In most homes, for example, the living room is set aside as a place of rest. The husband–patients' presence there reflected their felt need for a protective environment. Dens, finished basements, and attached work rooms, where the men might have chosen to repose in the days immediately following hospital discharge do not have the same symbolic value, nor would they have provided the same ready access to those who were performing nurse–surrogate roles.

Once men opted to become active, they changed location within the home. For example, now when he rested, Mr Ambrosio chose the den where he had a desk, and which was situated near the front door. He could bring in the mail and newspaper before his wife knew they had arrived. Seated at the front window he could greet his neighbors as they came home from work. He also could look out over his garden and mentally prepare his spring planting. Mr Stein likewise relocated from the living room to a corner off the kitchen where he stored the material he used to make stock market calculations. Responding to her husband's preference, Mrs Polski agreed to move the site of convalescence from the city to their country home. While these spatial changes were accompanied by some alteration in behavior, the symbolic value to the men of being in proximity to elements of their normal world underscores an important psychological shift in attitude toward physical activity.

These beginning steps, however small, radically altered the social and emotional climate in the homes. For the first time since prior to the illness, family conflict erupted. The wives and children, concerned and, in some cases, frightened, agreed that the men were displaying serious lack of judgement. They went to considerable lengths to halt the trend, including becoming uncharacteristically forceful. Mrs Stein, who it will be recalled, preferred to be noninvolved in her husband's affairs, became "hysterical" and "shrill" when she learned that her husband had smoked a cigarette at home. When she discovered that he stood on a chair to change a light bulb in the kitchen during her absence, she "hit the ceiling," and demanded that he not do such a thing in the future. Some tried physically to stop the men when they tried to carry out the garbage, or to walk out of doors. In so doing they were acting upon their felt obligation to control the patient's environment and prevent situations from occurring which would threaten his health and safety. The perspective of the husbands who were in fact apprehensive about what they could and could not safely accomplish was expressed by one of them this way:

> You just can't sit around for the rest of your life. I would not want to sit around for three months and all of a sudden start to move around. I don't believe that the doctors mean for you to do that anyway. They would rather see you move around gradually. That's my feeling on it anyway.

We see in this conflict the expression of differences in attitudes which originated during the earliest phase of hospitalization. The approach to activity of the husband–patients was in keeping with what they had experienced earlier. They saw the necessity to act and perceived dangers in extended passivity. Yet when they did so their uncertainty was apparent and was seized upon by spouses and children as a reason to postpone activity until such time as a safe course of action could be determined. They viewed such activity as misguided and an expression of impatience, tension, frustration, and the like; understandable but not worth the risks involved:

The things he is doing, it is just to do something. Doing the dishes, and I notice how he is eating. He used to be more relaxed . . . now he is eating and doesn't know what he is eating. I think he is very tense. He gets up and tries to do the dishes right away. He wants to do something, keep doing.

For the first time different perspectives on the nature of the illness and the requirements of care and treatment brought forth a confrontation between the spouses. Previously, different viewpoints existed but were not openly acknowledged. Patients and wives were not totally unaware that they held discrepant definitions of the situation, but the extent or basis of the differences were never explored.

The conflict over the activity of the husband–patient may also be conceived of as a struggle between conflicting claims to legitimacy in representing the medical point of view in the home. Each spouse felt more equipped than his or her partner to decide how best to give specific meaning in everyday terms to what the physician or nurse had said about "taking it easy." The husband–patients argued that their wives interpreted the medical regimen too strictly, while the wives felt they were morally obliged to prevent the men from engaging in what they perceived as potentially harmful behavior.

In pressing their respective claims for control of decision-making with regard to patient care, the spouses faced certain dilemmas. The wives saw themselves as essential to the preservation of the hospital-like atmosphere. They felt they could not simply withdraw from their role as medical surrogate. However, they realized that by continuing to insist that the men act as if they were still acutely ill, there was the very real possibility of upsetting them. This, in itself, would disturb their repose. For their part, the husbands had no way to demonstrate that they could safely perform the activities they were now proposing to do, and were not merely disobeying medical advice. There were no visible signs marking the transition from one state of health to another. They had no proof they were fit to leave the sick-role for one more compatible with rehabilitation. This is the reverse of a problem chronically ill patients in a later stage sometimes experience, that is, convincing persons unfamiliar with their condition, that they actually have a disabling condition – like heart disease – which, while it does not show, prevents them from full role participation (Kasselbaum and Baumann 1972).

In contrast to the earlier perception within the families that their troubles emanated from external sources, the present difficulties were seen to be directly related to ill-advised behavior of individuals inside the family. Thus, rather than closing ranks against an outside threat, the family members struggled with one another. The result was a noticeably decreased family harmony, in all the homes, and marked the beginning of a new stage in the family experience: The Early Period of Internal Stress.

Family Structure and Patterns of Rehabilitation Role Organization

While interpersonal conflict generated by discrepant expectations with regard to home-care role performance was a problem each of the families had to deal with shortly after the end of the *Period of Extension of Hospitalization*, the ways of problem solving varied according to important group values.

Adaptation to the current period of stress took three forms.

1 *Coercion*: Here family members attempted in various ways to force the husband–patient into compliance with the definition of the situation held by the wife and children.
2 *Disengagement*: Here, the strategy was to disengage from previous roles and to allow each person a greater share in decision-making responsibility, with no one person monopolizing the management of the home care.
3 *Reorganization*: Families in this case reached a mutually acceptable understanding that the wife would retain the major input into the organization of the recovery process.

Each mode of adaptation had a specific effect on the affective climate in the home. This outcome can be schematically represented in the following way:

Figure 1*

Time: *Stage one* ⟶	*Stage two*
(extension of	(strain and adjustment)
hospitalization)	
level of family	
integration – *consensus*	*reorganization*
period of	*disengagement*
conflict	*coercion*

* Variation on R. Hill (1958)[1]

Where *coercion* was the means used to settle differences with regard to home care behavior, affective relations between the husband–patient and others who now were his adversaries were marked by frequent hostility and antagonism. As defined by Spiegel (1957:403), coercion involves "manipulation of present and future punishments. Thus it ranges from overt attack to threats of attack in the future, and from verbal commands to physical force . . . If it is successful, the role conflict is settled through submission in which ego accepts the complimentary role enforced by alter." By attempting to coerce the husband into submitting to a role of seriously ill patient two negative consequences for the family sometimes surfaced: When the husband defied the others, conflict ensued; when he did submit, the result had alienation-like effects: the individual perceived that the family no longer fulfilled his goals or provided the outcomes he valued (Rosenstock and Kutner 1969).

Where family members choose to *disengage* from previously held role definitions, each party accepted somewhat less autonomy than he or she desired. Something like Spiegel's (1957:407) concept "role reversal" seemed to apply whereby "ego proposes that alter put himself in ego's shoes, trying to see things through his eyes." This was a pragmatic attempt to stabilize relationships which had become conflict-ridden due to discordant role expectations. However, stress was still present because each person was behaving in less than complete harmony with his or her desires.

Where *reorganization* occurred, family members experienced a heightened sense of togetherness. Spiegel (1957:402) uses the term "role modification" for this situation, meaning that "the change in role expectations is bilateral, and modification techniques are based on interchanges and mutual identifications of ego with alter." In this case, the wife was able to fully actualize her expectations with regard to her and her husband's home-care role behavior. The husband, in this stage of his patient career, was willing to accept a strong nurse-surrogate role on the part of his spouse.

Disengagement: The Mode of Adaptation in Divergent Families

Although it is difficult to know precisely when and how the disengagement mode of adaptation began, it appears that the first steps to reduce the hostility were taken by the wives, who diminished the level of their opposition to their husband's behavior and disengaged, in part, from the nurse–surrogate role. Each backed off from the initial expectation of full control.

Mrs Stein who had earlier described her response to some of her husband's behavior as "shrill" and "like a shrew" explained that she could just not cope with the ill feeling generated by her attempts to coerce her husband. Besides, she felt it was having a negative influence on her own physical and emotional health, as well. Her husband, Mr Stein, described the change in her approach: "On certain things I get bawled out. I mean endearingly."

In place of strident arguing, these four wives turned to persuasion as a means of influencing their husband's behavior. They also compromised. For example, if Mr Asti firmly stated his intention to descend the basement steps, his wife only insisted that he go very slowly, support himself on the railing, and allow her to help. The Asti's daughter, Rose, explained that since her father became angry whenever anyone tried to interfere with his plans, her response was to be helpful but not interfering. She explained: "I would not keep asking: 'Do you want this, or this, or this?' I would just do what is necessary." In other words, she remained involved, but at a judicious distance.

The wives tried to remain vigilant of their husbands, often suggesting that they rest or postpone some activity until a later time. I asked Mr Polski, shortly after he and his wife had gone to their country home, how often his wife reminded him to slow down his pace. He replied, "Well, she leaves that up to me. But she's after me. Like I wanted to do a little but this morning she said: 'Don't knock yourself out.' She was after me from three o'clock to knock it off, because the day before I had gotten chest pains."

By remaining close at hand, wives not only hoped to persuade the men to do less, but actually to assist them and thus lessen the burden of activity. Mrs Polski explained: "Yesterday he was rushing around so much, I swept the basement so he could get done quicker. If he does it, he'll never come up." Mrs Warren, who before the illness rarely engaged in joint activity with her husband, now sat with him so she could be available to perform small services like turning the TV dial, bringing in the newspaper, getting a cup of tea.

Mrs Asti learned that while sometimes she could assist her husband with his activities, there was also the chance that her actions would be interpreted as interference and lead to quarreling. Therefore, she began to ask relatives to "drop by" when her husband was planning to make some household repair and provide some assistance. He was less able to refuse offers of help from others. However, in order to utilize this strategy most effectively, Mrs Asti had to follow her husband's activities closely. While she tried to be non-interfering they both realized that she remained highly aware of his whereabouts, and plans.

In playing a modified nurse–surrogate role, the wife was still able to communicate her views to the man and was a restraining influence on his behavior.

In each of these divergent families there was evidence that the husband–patients felt obliged to respect wifely advice. Moreover, the men indicated that this input could be valuable in preventing them from misjudging their real limitations. Mr Polski said: "I think it is good to have my wife reminding me of what to do rather than have someone who didn't care. If she didn't, I'd probably be doing something I shouldn't. It's like in the hospital where you have a nurse after you all the time." While the patient–husbands perceived their limitations in a less restrictive fashion than their wives did, most were still convinced they had a serious medical problem; one which could become dangerously worse if they over-exerted themselves. They were willing to be active, and even test the limits of their present strength, but doubts about their health, and uncertainty about recovery still remained. Prior to his first medical examination since leaving the hospital, Mr Asti commented: "I want to ask if there is any difference in my physical being; if I'm doing alright. Am I coming along as expected or not?" When I asked how he thought he was doing at this point he replied: "I have no way of knowing." This was doubtlessly instrumental in his susceptibility to persuasion by wife and children. When I asked about his decision to go outside the house for the first time he replied: "My wife didn't want me to do anything. So, being the doctor said take it easy, I figured I'd let another week go by before I tried anything else."

In contrast to those occasions when wifely admonition would cause a man to reevaluate his intended behavior from the standpoint of his own safety, there were times when he seemed to agree with her solely out of respect for her feelings. On a number of occasions, when asked to give examples of disagreements the men had with their wives over how to interpret the medical regimen, the men would describe occasions on which they started to do some activity but stopped after wives raised objections. When asked to explain, they might reply: "Oh, what's the use of arguing," or "I don't know, I just didn't bother."

Willingness occasionally to adhere to the perspective of the wife, along with tolerating her constant advice and admonition, also seemed to be the reciprocal response of the husband–patient to his wife's disengagement from actively seeking a controlling nurse-surrogate role in the home care. It recognized the right of the wife to have some input into the recovery process, without controlling it. It gave her a sense of responsibility, and allowed her to feel successful in carrying out her felt obligations to keep the man from hazardous circumstances. Without some input into the home care, the wife might have no option but to demand a share in decision making, precipitating a hostile response. It also left the patient–husband fairly free to choose when to comply with the wife's interpretation of the medical regimen.

On the other hand, the men could be forceful in rejecting wifely attempts to control their behavior. They only selectively followed their wife's counsel. Concerning his smoking, Mr Stein demanded that his wife leave it to him to deal with. He told her that it was something he would handle in his own way. He never attempted to conceal the fact of his smoking. Openness, rather than subterfuge was characteristic of men in divergent households. They did not pretend to others that they were doing less than they actually were.

Limitations in the strategy of disengagement were evident particularly when the wives perceived the men's activity as especially arduous, or when the men had episodes of angina. This would compel the wives to act forcefully in pressing their opinion on the men. The spectre of marital conflict made this a difficult choice, as Mrs Stein's statement clearly demonstrates:

> When we get to the doctor at the center, there is a tremendous walk from where he parks the car to the doctor. Will he be able to maneuver that, will he be able to manage it? Should I call in advance and have somebody meet him there with a wheelchair or something? I don't know if he will want that. He's apt to blast me with his tongue out of creation.

Another source of stress to the family members during this stage of adjustment, which points up a further limitation of the disengagement mode of dealing with problems, was the fact that the real depth of personal concern was not shared. The husband who felt discomfiture in his chest did not feel free to express his concern to his wife or children; lest they feel obliged to intervene. In order not to add to the patient's problems, wives and children deliberately refrained from revealing the full extent of their own fears and doubts.

Against the remarkable similarities in their ways of handling the immediate post-hospital days and subsequent shifts, there were, of course, individual differences in levels of group tension, conflict, and disorganization. Factors associated with adaptation in divergent families were the perception within the home of the state of the patient–husband's health; and the fit between the nurse-like role the wife was able to play and her perception of her husband's need for external control.

If the patient appeared to be showing signs of improving health and was taking some precautions, a limited nurse-like role was sufficient for the wife, who, in keeping with normal family preferences was not used to imposing her will on others in the family. She could begin to pursue activities that normally provided important satisfaction in her life. Likewise, the husband could begin to resume some familiar activities that were important to him. On the other hand declining health, or even lack of perception of improvement, tended to produce marital discord and intrapersonal stress because the wife was not satisfied that her efforts on the patient's behalf were sufficient to produce the desired healthful atmosphere in the home.

During this stage, The Early Period of Internal Stress, the Polski's experienced the least disruption of normal routines, and interpersonal relationships. Shortly after Mr and Mrs Polski returned to their country home, he began doing what he described as "light work." This involved cleaning up, sorting his tools, etc. He was, however, taking two naps a day, something he rarely did before the illness. When he experienced any pain in his chest he took a nitroglycerine tablet and stopped working. Significantly, both attributed discomfiture to his need for rest, not to any abnormality in the heart itself. In other words, they believed he was progressing normally. The pain was perceived as a warning to stop working, not an inherent danger sign in and of itself. Their confidence in his improvement seemed to be justified by his increasing tolerance for work. By the second week he was able both to increase the length of time he could work and to do more strenuous labor: he cut his naps down to one and worked until 4.30. On weekends he and his wife began to resume a bit of socializing. On these occasions, he found then that he could violate the dietary requirements without any noticeable after-effects.

Mrs Polski continued to remind her husband about the

need for caution and restraint, but she did not often feel obliged to challenge him, or press her viewpoint against his wishes. She said that although it troubled her when he took nitroglycerine, he seemed to be getting stronger, and this tempered her disapproval of his activities. Several times she began telling of projects she tried to discourage, only to say eventually, "Well, I can see his point too."

Because of this perception, Mrs Polski felt free to pursue many of her own activities. When asked: "How about yourself, are you as busy as you normally are?" she replied,

Oh yes, I don't know where the day goes – I can't understand how some women can say they are lonesome, or they are bored. I could never say that. I can't seem to catch up. I have so much to do. I'm either knitting something or fixing something. The day is not long enough to accomplish what I want. My husband is the same way. The days go so fast.

When asked: "Is your routine the same or different than before your husband became ill?" she replied, "The same. It is just the same."

Even the fact that she was not taking her normal trips into the city to visit her friends and go to club meetings did not seem to cause her very much disappointment. She accepted this limitation on her freedom as part of her obligation to her husband during his recovery. She felt she had a role to play in reminding him to be cautious and in helping him with his chores. She anticipated that without her presence, Mr Polski would tend to do more than he was doing at present. She felt she had an effective voice in the recovery process.

On each of the factors outlined above, the Polski's measured up favorably. Mr Polski's health was perceived as growing better steadily. In spite of occasional excesses, it seemed to his wife that he did demonstrate a willingness to change normal behavior in favor of more cautious "sick role behavior," which was consonant with his perceived health status. His wife was able to play a nurse role she felt was adequate in view of his needs, and was still able to pursue her own activities.

At the opposite end of the spectrum of response in the

Second Stage were the Steins. Interpersonal relations were uncharacteristically strained and there was a good deal of individual emotional stress. Each spouse was disappointed with the role behavior of the other. There were regular conflicts which created an atmosphere of tension in the home. Hostility was ignited easily.

Mr Stein began to have chest pain soon after returning from the hospital. Pain, sometimes intense, came without exertion, and both partners were, not surprisingly, concerned about this. After several days home he began to violate aspects of the medical regimen in blatant ways. For one thing he resumed smoking, and, in a further violation of medical orders, drove to the store to get his cigarettes. In doing so, Mr Stein made no attempt to hide this fact from his wife who associated smoking with the heart attack. Mr Stein, himself, called what he was doing, "my own form of suicide." His wife, bitterly opposed to his actions, accused him of "driving nails into your coffin."

Her reaction to his behavior was a combination of frustration at not being able to control events and dreaded anticipation of continuous conflict which was the cost of taking the aggressive stance she felt was required of her. Caught by conflicting needs, the couple had unusually frequent arguments and periods of somber withdrawal.

An additional factor behind Mr Stein's refusal to allow all but a minimal nurse role for his wife was that he believed she did not have sufficient knowledge to make decisions affecting his care. She made what he called "bad judgement mistakes." Examples he gave of this included inviting relatives to visit when he was not feeling well, and, particularly, her lack of adequacy in the area of food preparation. Prior to his illness her lack of cooking skills were a source of amusement. Now, because the diet was the part of the regimen Mr Stein valued most, it became a source of antagonism. His wife remarked on this problem: "Now when I come home I get arguments from him: 'What supper are you going to ruin tonight? What are you going to feed me tonight that I am not going to like? What chemicals are you going to give me tonight?' I never had that with him before." Although Mr Stein began to seek out information himself on matters such as nutritional supplements, and recipes for cooking the bland food he was now required to eat, his wife did not become involved in this task. In interviews, she acknowledged her lack of information and blamed this on the medical staff at the hospital:

I haven't been told a thing about what to expect: physically, sexually, or brainwise. On TV it said that sex is the best thing after a heart attack. How do I know that's so? Suppose he gets an attack when we are having relations? What then? I don't even know who his doctor is that took care of him in the hospital. [E.S.: "What gives you the idea that he can't for example walk out on the porch and take the air?"] I don't know. I have no idea. (Yet she was opposed to this activity.)

What was especially upsetting to Mrs Stein was that during the first week at home life had been pleasant. Her advice was accepted and her cooking tolerated. She longed for a return to the easy tranquility the couple had known when together in the past.

Since coming home from the hospital, Mr Stein was beset with a series of upsetting experiences: pain, fevers, flu symptoms. He fought depression by trying to become involved in his hobbies, and doing some chores around the house. "I don't want them thinking of me as an invalid," he declared in reference to his wife and married daughter. "I'm taking a positive approach. I'm looking ahead to getting back to work." At worst, he looked upon his wife's attempts to play a nurse role as detrimental to his recovery. Most of the time he just thought she could not contribute much. I asked him: "How much is your wife involved in your activities at home?" He replied simply: "What can she do?"

The experience of the Asti family in coping with home care adjustments fell between the two that I have just described. Mr Asti did not have chest pain or take nitroglycerine, but he still considered himself in fragile health. He tended to be cautious, and unsure of himself. Yet he was willing to begin some minor activities, even though he worried as he did them. Lack of confidence in his recovery made him tense and unsure of how to go about what he thought was required of him: i.e., gradually increasing activities. He was anxiously awaiting news of his condition.

For weeks, he only attempted to do small chores like drying

the dishes, carrying garbage bags to the pail, picking up papers from the yard. His wife was inclined to try to discourage most of these activities. He said that he often had to tell her: "I feel alright. I want to do it now. I can't sit down for the rest of my life." He did however, let her help him in some of these activities.

Mrs Asti had more of a substantial role in managing the convalescence than did either Mrs Polski or Mrs Stein. She was completely in charge of the preparation of the food. She claimed that the hospital did not provide her with a diet to follow, so she developed her own set of guidelines, by remembering what he was given to eat in the hospital. Her other resources were her own "weight watchers" diet, and the diabetic diet her own mother had been on. Mr Asti seemed pleased that his wife was handling this and in matters related to food, he gave his wife full recognition. For example, he often said things like, "My wife is trying to keep me on a low calorie diet as much as possible." Or, "My wife thinks I ought to lose some weight." He also seemed to rely on her to remind him of when to take his medication. Prior to his heart attack, he had been diagnosed as a diabetic, but had stopped taking the medication when he felt better. Now, he was using his wife to insure against this happening again. In contrast to the previous example, Mr Asti perceived his wife as competent in at least this important aspect of his recovery.

It was evident during this period that each of the members of the family was making an effort to avoid confrontation. Rose said she tried to be helpful around the house, and during this time did more chores to help her mother than she normally did. Mrs Asti appeared adept at knowing when she could express her own opinions about the medical care requirements, and when she should maintain her distance from her husband's affairs. For his part, Mr Asti tolerated suggestions, and when he did not want interference, generally was firm but non-hostile.

Yet occasions when the members clashed could not be avoided completely. Balancing a sense of obligation to have the patient–husband do less, with strongly held family norms of noninterference and individual autonomy, created tensions. At times Mrs Asti could not restrain her need to express her views forcefully, and sought support for her position from her daughter. However, Rose did not agree. In contrast to her earlier stance it became Rose's opinion that her father should be left to follow his own inclinations. Occasionally this different approach to the problem created heated exchanges between mother and daughter.

Aside from occasional episodes of interpersonal conflict, most of the tension in the Asti family was intrapersonal. Neither Mr or Mrs Asti was comfortable resuming normal activities, and as a consequence, were often in each other's presence. Prior to the illness, Mrs Asti spent many afternoons with her friends. Now she mainly stayed at home to be near her husband. Seeing him do more than she thought was wise upset her. Yet she knew that she had to be judicious about expressing opposition to his activities. The novelty of having his actions scrutinized by his wife was something Mr Asti tolerated but did not enjoy. In spite of being in close proximity for long periods of time, the couple did not seem to develop more of an active companionship.

If we examine the adjustments made in the second stage of the home care in the light of pre-illness family patterns, certain explanations for this coping style suggest themselves. Individuals ordinarily expected to have much discretion in the performance of their daily activities. Social organization allowed for flexibility in role performance. This was related to the high value placed on separation, as opposed to togetherness, both in activity in the home as well as in activity with external groups and interests.

For a short time after hospital discharge, a role differentiated division of labor prevailed in each of these homes. Separation from the hospital temporarily constrained the husband–patients to seek a sense of security in a passive–dependent patient role and encouraged wives and children to assume highly dominant nurse–surrogate roles. However, as soon as the husbands regained a sense of security in their surroundings, their preference for deciding for themselves what daily activities should consist of asserted itself. After a period of struggle, the couples, recognizing a need to adopt a strategy to mediate their interpersonal conflicts, attempted to strike a new balance based on mutual participation without interference. Wives continued to give advice, but withdrew from active opposition in the face of continued insistance on the part of the men to behave according to their own needs and interpretation of the regimen. The husband–patients in various ways recognized the right of wives to participate in the home care management. In effect, the couple attempted to fit the management of the recovery to the pre-illness pattern: each person participates, neither is excluded, but the norm of noninterference in personal choice necessitates that the husband–patient has the final word in determining his own behavior.

For the wife to have continued to act as if it were her role alone to manage the recovery process, she would have acted in a nonprecedented way given the family's structure and value climate. She would have risked upsetting the basis on which marital stability rested had she tried to impose a role differentiated order in a family which valued role exchange. It was no more in the wife's interest to do this, than it was for the husband. Being a full-time nurse–surrogate would have increased the chances of marital disharmony with no corresponding rewards. In other words, there were no social gains to be had for the wife by increasing her control over her husband's behavior. She did not gain by increasing her role in the family, nor did she value the closeness which a husband–patient, wife–nurse relationship would bring. On the contrary, what she valued was her own independence and her own separate lifestyle.

Home Care Adjustment In Convergent and Discordant Families

The advantages and limitations of the disengagement mode of problem solving are exemplified in the case histories presented above. While consistent with family values, its fit with the everyday requirements of home-based recovery from heart attack was more problematic. The promise it offered of achieving a balance between the needs of the recovering heart patient and the psychosocial wellbeing of the conjugal unit was not always fulfilled, and in one case, was thoroughly shattered.

In other families, wives responded to the husband–patients' attempts to increase autonomous behavior with more, not less, intense and active opposition of their own. Their efforts withstood a short period of challenge by the men who, for the next six to eight weeks, had their activities supervised and planned by others in the family. While not always in agreement, they seemed to accept the dominant role of wife and child in the home care.

In two cases, involving Mr O'Shea and Mr Goldberg, the men returned home from the hospital very fearful and confused. Mr O'Shea believed he was better off in the hospital than he was at home and for weeks did little more than sleep or sit by the window in his pajamas. Before either man attempted any activity, he checked with his wife. An active wife–nurse was desired by these two men.

In contrast, Mr Grasso and Mr Ambrosio accepted control of their behavior by others in the family less willingly. Yet, for the most part, they complied with the direction given by the wives and/or children. Mr Grasso "argued over terms," but usually Mrs Grasso's interpretation of the regimen prevailed. Mr Ambrosio sometimes objected to the restrictions his wife placed on him. He gave the following example:

> So we folded the laundry and put them in the position she wanted them and that was it. But she wouldn't let me take the basket up [here, he slammed his hand on the table]. See, to me this is wrong, I just feel that sooner or later I'm just going to do it and she won't say boo. [His voice rises in anger.]

Nevertheless, it was over a month before Mr Ambrosio would openly challenge her authority in these matters.

The four men in convergent and discordant relationships seemed to rely on their wives' knowledge of the medical regimen. Explaining why he refrained from going out of doors, Mr Grasso explained: "Well, I think it would be alright. My wife seems to feel that the doctor says I should stay in the house. She remembers my routine should be confined inside the house." Mr Ambrosio, in response to a similar question, answered "I knew she was being briefed all the time she was in that hospital. She would be getting Dr J.'s ear [the medical director of Group Hospital] or whoever's ear she could grab." Mrs O'Shea, when asked why her spouse followed her advice now, since before the illness he often did not, explained, "I'm known as the doctor without the shingle in this family."

Mr Grasso and Mr Ambrosio did increase their activities somewhat during the weeks following homecoming. But they were not as active as their counterparts. Moreover, the kinds of activities they performed were, for the most part, unrelated to their former role activities. Mr Ambrosio channeled his activities into crafts like painting, ceramics, hooking rugs. At his wife's urging, Mr O'Shea did not call his friends on the phone. Likewise, Mrs Grasso insisted that her husband not examine the records or daily receipts of their business or to help plan the purchasing for the store during this period. She and her son Anthony assumed these functions entirely. The O'Shea family was in the midst of preparing for their daughter's wedding when the heart attack struck. Mrs O'Shea and her daughter, not wanting him "to get excited," insisted that he refrain from involving himself with planning for the event. She and her daughter assumed this entire function. All claimed that under normal circumstances, he would have been involved a great deal.

For a period which lasted up to two months, the wives, with the help of children, made almost all the decisions with regard to the care, and handled all family business. As a consequence, husbands in convergent and discordant families were less active, and farther away from resuming normal social functions than were the others at the same point in time.

Wives especially carried out their expanded functions, with exceptional zeal. The claim they made to full control of the nurse function was compatible with the normal family values and lifestyle (or that which wives had been pushing for before the illness). That is, when any task is assigned, it is expected to become the responsibility of a particular family member. Others are obliged to reciprocate with appropriate behavior of their own. These reciprocal roles and obligations are ordinarily not interchangeable among the family members. When after hospitalization, the task of patient supervision fell to the wife, she did not expect to share it with her husband. Change in the balance of influence over family affairs brought opportunities for social gain. This is due to the fact that the family was the major source of need fulfillment and emotional gratification for the members who had an interest in making the behavior of others congruent with their own expectations. Being a nurse–surrogate, the wife could now organize the day-to-day family life so that even more than before the illness it was compatible with her own interests and aspirations. Normally, she shared control over the content of family life with her husband. Both had their own spheres of influence which made them interdependent. In some areas of their life together, there had been disagreement and disharmony. Now the wife had a chance to alter the patterns she found particularly disagreeable.

The wives who had the most to gain by controlling the recovery were the two from discordant families – Mrs Ambrosio and Mrs O'Shea. Their pre-illness disappointments over the content of home life had been great. In contrast to their present positions before the illness, they had little success at influencing their husband's behavior.

An indication of how successful their wives were in establishing the legitimacy of their claim to home care control was that when husbands did deviate from wives instructions they did so *in secret*. When the couple was together, the husband–patient sometimes complained but almost never went directly against his wife's wishes. The wives were prepared to act forcefully to meet any deviation from their policies, and the men reported that they were aware of the conflict that could follow when they did not follow orders. This is illustrated by the following exchange between Mr Ambrosio and the interviewer:

> (Interviewer) I saw that big branch was gone. (Mr Ambrosio) I have a saw. No sweat, only I had to do it when she wasn't around. (Interviewer) I guess she noticed. (Mr Ambrosio) No, and I haven't said a word either. [I did it] Little by little . . . it could have led to a divorce.

Along with the similarities I have described, the emotional climate during this second stage of home care was not the

same for the discordant families as it was for the Grasso's
where prior to the illness both spouses actively supported a
role differentiated family structure. While elements of coer-
sion were present in both convergent and discordant homes
during the period we are addressing, this mode of adaptation
lasted longer in the Grasso family. In the two discordant
homes, Mr Ambrosio and Mr O'Shea adopted attitudes of
restraint and passivity which are consistent with the sick role.
Ironically, couples who prior to the illness were unable to
reach a consensus on conjugal roles managed to do so during
the initial stages of home care.

The Honeymoon Period in Discordant Families –
Reorganization in the Ambrosio and O'Shea Families

The restrictions the regimen placed on the men and which
their spouses reinforced brought immediate gains to the
wives. Mrs Ambrosio explained it this way: "I always felt my
husband did many things that I could do that he wouldn't let
me do, and I feel so stupid in so many things. I feel that now
he should let me." She took over as many household chores as
she could manage to do: food shopping everyday, even
though there are only two of them, preparing all the meals and
then doing the dishes, shopping for her husband's clothing
and selecting what he would wear during the day – all things
which she wanted to do before but could not because her
husband did them first. She was finally in control of the
household. Whenever I saw or spoke to her during the weeks
of the second stage, she appeared happy and spoke en-
thusiastically of her daily routine: "I never felt better in my
life. [My younger sister] is always saying on the phone: 'Are
you resting? Are you resting?' But when the came she said:
'My God, you look wonderful.' " The chores she was so happy
doing were "wifely" chores, ones which prior to the illness
she wanted to be in charge of. "It's a nice feeling getting up
early, it's dark, and I get the breakfast ready, put the shades
up to let the light in. *Then I wait on him.*" Mr Ambrosio
was both surprised and impressed with his wife's energy. He
told me:

Like this morning, she said she got up at 4 am. I said,

"What the hell did you get up at four?" She said "I want the floor washed." "I really want to know why you get up so early, what is the advantage?" I'm suddenly finding out: it is peaceful, quiet, there is no interruption, telephone or other duties.

Mrs O'Shea reported the same type of rewarding experience during this part of the home care. She was able to actualize her wishes for an orderly home, in which activities followed a definite routine:

We eat on time now. My life doesn't revolve around the Knights of Columbus, or anybody. It revolves around me . . . I hated that. I wanted to eat at a certain time, I'd get a phone call [from her husband] "I'll be a half hour late," and a half hour would go into an hour. . . I got like a hound dog . . . I have the say now. I don't get, "Well this is my job. . . if you don't want to wait, don't wait . . ." Everything is me, what I have to say, no more what he has to say . . . Now [he says] what do *you* think, not: "I'm going to do it this way."

Both women utilized the inability of their husbands to participate outside of the home to increase their own closeness – to substitute themselves for their husband's separate friends and interests. This was something these women had wanted to accomplish prior to the illness but could not. Before, Mrs Ambrosio and Mrs O'Shea were denied it, but now the situation enabled them to have it. Mrs O'Shea related: "I was always around. Now I have a companion. It is better for me . . . It is for my benefit for a change. He checks the programs for us to watch . . . We talk back and forth. Normally, I would be staring at the television with no one to talk to." Mrs Ambrosio, who had a very active life outside the family prior to the illness, ceased all of these involvements and was glad of it. She claimed that what she was doing now at home pleased her more than church and community activities. She liked reading to her sick husband, talking with him, helping him with his hobbies, and most of all providing nurturance and service.

Mrs O'Shea's advice to her husband seemed designed to separate him from those external forces that she blamed for his separation from the family. She blamed his friends, "bad

guys" she called them, for his past neglect of her wishes and
now during the convalescence she used her influence to make
his medical condition appear incompatible with his former
friends and activities. She discouraged his friends from
visiting him. She told me: "I have not let anybody come up
here. He will want to be the host . . . If friends do come I'm
not afraid to say, 'Jim has to go to bed now'; or 'I can't allow
smoking around Jim now.'" Yet, at the same time, she
portrayed them to her husband as unfaithful friends. "People
he was very friendly with have never called. I say, 'I told you
so, I never liked that person.' Then I'm in my glory."

When Mr O'Shea began to feel well enough to go out for
brief walks, Mrs O'Shea sometimes used who he was likely to
meet as her criteria for approving or discouraging the activity.
For example, her argument against his going to church
service was: "You know everybody is going to talk to you. It
isn't that you are going to go and come back, everybody will
grab you in the back of the church." On the other hand,
during this same period, she encouraged him to go to a
wedding of her relatives, even though he said he did not feel
up to it. In this case, she argued that "talking to people will do
him good." In other words, she encouraged him in activities
that they would do together, and discouraged him from those
that involved his friends. She substituted for his friends.

In time Mr O'Shea began to look forward to his wife's
company. When his wife came home from work he was
openly glad to see her and, in a switch of patterns, got angry if
his wife went out in the evening to visit her friends. As the
rehabilitation progressed, closeness between Mr and Mrs
O'Shea increased markedly. They developed a new ritual. In
the afternoon, as soon as he saw her step off the bus (he looked
out the window around the time she should be arriving), he
would start brewing a pot of tea and make her a snack. Then
they would eat and talk. He started driving at his wife's
urging – she needed to be driven home from her daughter's
shower. This was prior to the doctor giving approval for this
activity. For several weeks thereafter he picked her up from
work in the afternoon and then drove her shopping. Formerly, she did these chores alone.

One of the reasons why Mr Ambrosio was pleased to have

his wife close by was that he perceived her as having a positive effect on his progress toward health. Mr Ambrosio admitted that even though there were times he wanted to disagree with his wife and do more than she allowed, "She is right in many respects." He seemed pleasantly surprised at how much she could accomplish around the house, and how adroitly she managed his care. His wife reflected on his sentiments during the first month of the home care: "I think he has a little more confidence in what I'm doing . . . He told me he owes his life to me. In letters he writes, people tell me: I give him tender loving care. If it wasn't for me he wouldn't have made it."

Under her supervision, Mr Ambrosio felt confident that his health was improving. He said: "I've learned what foods to eat . . . I can feel an infusion of energy into my body. Because now for the first time I'm eating like I should be eating . . . I would have pancakes piled up to here. Clara would not follow through. Now, if I do she is right on me with a baseball bat."

Neither Mr O'Shea or Mr Ambrosio gave indications that their present passive role challenged the security of their self images. In the normal course of their day-to-day lives prior to the illness, neither person was concerned about sex role boundaries. Both were willing – even anxious – to do activities traditionally ascribed to females in our society. Having their wives temporarily substituting for them was not intrinsically threatening to them. Mr Ambrosio reflected on the role that his wife was currently playing, and seemed willing to accept the change in their relationship, at least for the present.

She said like a school teacher: "Don't you worry about a thing, you just do as you are told" (E.S.: Is that something characteristic of her to give you an admonition like that?) No, there it points out – I think this is characteristic of all women – the motherly instinct comes out. Not the wifely instinct, per se. First the motherly instinct: "You are the little person, you are sick and I have to treat you like an invalid . . . and you are going to listen to me."

With Mr O'Shea not working, the financial burden of the family was the sole responsibility of Mrs O'Shea. While the decrease in income troubled Mr O'Shea, the fact that he was not the family breadwinner was not in itself a problem to him. He hoped that the promotion and raise his wife was scheduled for would make him less worried about the family's finances. It also pleased him very much when his married son offered to give him a sum of money whenever he needed it.

Comparing life in the Ambrosio family during the second stage of home care with what it had been like before the illness, one cannot fail to notice the remarkable improvement in the wife's morale and self image. Moreover, the marital relationship itself was noticeably more harmonious. There was little of the former arguing between the spouses over who should take responsibility for household tasks. Mr Ambrosio, for the most part, appeared willing to play a passive patient role, which he perceived as necessary for full recovery later on. Occasionally, he verbalized impatience, and even acted against his wife's wishes by going to the mailbox in the rain or walking farther than she wanted. But when his wife corrected him, he resumed a compliant posture without becoming hostile. His wife seemed to thrive on nurturing him. She liked reading poetry to him, selecting what clothing he should wear, and what and when he should eat.

It is difficult to exaggerate Mrs Ambrosio's happiness over her role. Doing everyday mundane chores seemed to delight her. After she salted down the sidewalk after a frost, she remarked to her husband and me that she felt like a young girl on her parents' farm feeding the chickens. With a sense of self discovery she discussed a book she had just read about the positive aspects of being middle aged. "It is truly wonderful," she exclaimed.

In spite of present harmony, there were some signs that the future would not be as harmonious as the present in the Ambrosio household. Mr Ambrosio perceived the present state of affairs as temporary. I asked him if he thought he would ever again resume all of his former activities, many of which his wife was now taking delight in. "Oh yeah, I want it that way. This is my job . . . This I expect to do. I know damn well that she will literally have to hold me down . . . these things I want to do myself; take the car out, take the garbage, go shopping . . ." This was not the impression Mrs Ambrosio conveyed, however. While she did not expect to continue to do quite as much as she was now, she perceived the illness as having brought a permanent change in the marital relationship. Her understanding of the consequences of the heart attack was that the husband would never be able to go back to a highly active lifestyle. She recalled that one of his doctors had told her he would never be able to do anything as strenuous as changing a tire on his car. The couple, however, never discussed future adjustments. They concentrated their interaction on the present.

The Burden and the Promise of Coercive Role Adjustment – The Grassos

The experience of the Grasso family demonstrates that the second stage of home care can be a troubled time for a family, in spite of the increase in control by the wife.

Mr Grasso was displeased by the restrictions on his activities, and he particularly resented being subject to the authority of his wife and son. He argued, complained, and criticized the present state of affairs. Mrs Grasso, however, was unrelenting in her insistence on making all the decisions regarding her husband's activity. In the past when she tried to influence others' behavior, she did so in a quiet way. Now, however, she pressed her position, and argued, as she said, in "an unladylike way." She told me: "I nag him all the time: What did you eat? Are you allowed? Did you go down the stairs? He gets annoyed, but that's how I play my role."

Having his wife and son plan and operate the family business and do his household chores bothered Mr Grasso. He felt deeply about his masculine breadwinner role and was unable to adjust to a passive patient role, which he felt was humiliating. He said to me one day: "It used to be that she waited by the window for me to come home. Now, I'm waiting for her to come home. It is not easy . . . I'm not being chauvinistic, but it is not easy for a man to do."

Anthony was ambivalent about the role he felt obliged to play in the home now. Criticizing his father's behavior seemed out of character even though he felt it was needed. His father gave an illustration of his son's conflict: "I lit a cigarette the other day. I shouldn't and he caught me smoking. He chewed me out as much as a son would dare to chew a father out. He was embarrassed." (E.S.: Why was he embarrassed?) "The fact that he caught me doing something wrong. He walked out of the room, mad, but he didn't say anything angry to me. I felt so bad; I threw the cigarette away immediately." The requirements of illness had altered the basic structure of parent–child relations. Father and son both disliked it. Anthony and his father had always formed a coalition in which they attempted to influence the direction of certain family matters to which Mrs Grasso was opposed. The strong bond between father and son was something each family member reported. Anthony seemed especially gratified by it. However, his present role in the rehabilitation was stressful to him because it resulted in a coalition between mother and son vis à vis father. Yet, Anthony felt that this was what the situation required.

Mr Grasso, in describing his first trip to the doctor since homecoming, illustrated his new isolated position in the family:

> Anthony came with me, not so much for company, but I think for – they play games with me. They want to be sure I don't lie to them, if when I ask the doctor if I can go to the store [business] I would say yes, when in fact he had said no. My wife feels that I abuse the doctor's warnings. I'm pretty sure that's the only reason Anthony was there.

Unlike many of the other men at this time, Mr Grasso had serious doubts about ever getting well – even if he conformed to a very conservative regimen. He stated:

> But somehow I feel that sometime I'll go back there again, not with a terminal attack, but I'll have reason to go back to the hospital with some kind of heart attack again . . . one of the doctors said it . . . my wife thought that was very silly but I don't think it was silly. I feel that way . . . whatever conditions put me there the first time still prevail and it is not a matter of eating too much chocolates or smoking too many cigars either. It's just a condition that is within my constitution that just does not leave by cutting out sugar and smoking."

At home he did stop smoking (for a short time at least) and for the first three weeks generally followed Mrs Grasso's advice, although with reluctance. He said in our first talk at home, "I feel very well, very good, just restless. I feel strong enough. I have no worry about being able to walk a block or two. I'm afraid because the doctors didn't say that I could. I'm trying to do the right thing. Whether or not I think it is right or wrong I guess doesn't matter." Moments later, he indicated that he felt a responsibility to cooperate with his family whom he saw as suffering because of his illness. "I say the problem, whatever put me there, will never be cured . . . I can't change that by eating different. I'm trying to be calm. I'm going to try to change. *I promised. I owe it to them to change.*"

Without this felt obligation to subordinate his own preferences to the demands of the group, which is required under the values of convergence, Mr Grasso's rejection of the institutional definitions and prescribed procedures to cure, control or minimize the effects of the illness would probably have led to a "retreatist" behavioral response. Merton (1968:242) defines the retreatist mode of adaptation as follows:

> Retreatism seems to occur in response to acute anomie, involving an abrupt break in the familiar and accepted normative framework and in established social relations, particularly when it appears to individuals subjected to it that the condition will continue indefinitely . . . it often obtains in those patterned situations which "exempt" individuals from a wide array of role obligations, as, for example, in the case of "retirement" from the job imposed upon people without their consent . . .

Yet, Mr Grasso made an effort to conform to a set of expected behaviors even though he failed to see the usefulness of them, and experienced psychological stress in carrying them out. The evidence is that the weight of the family's collectivity orientation created a sense of obligation on the part of the patient to conform with the expectations of the group. However, the discontinuity between his subjective feelings and the demands of social obligation made conformity difficult, and there were lapses in it. His inner tension was expressed in aggressiveness, anger toward his wife and son, and depression – all of which contributed to the overall family climate during the second stage of home care.

In playing her role, Mrs Grasso had to deal with these tensions. Anger on her husband's part did not diminish the extent of her attention to the details – large and small – of his care. She determined whether the doctor's order to rest at home meant that the husband could not sit on the porch in the sun for a few moments. She determined when he was able to see his friends, and to join in the card games. To her husband's chagrin she even answered for him when friends inquired about his treatment regimen.

According to Mr Grasso, his wife derived a measure of satisfaction over her success in controlling his behavior. With friends, she discussed her role, and he listened in: "You overhear: 'Is he resting' 'Yes, I won't let him do anything. He wants to go outside. He wants to work. I won't let him,' my wife would say proudly. She refused to let me outside, and its a feather in her cap."

Mrs Grasso paid a personal price for her nurse role. She reported that overseeing her husband's care left her little time for much else. She was up late doing housework. When she came home from work she had to do the bookkeeping for the store and the planning for the next day. She was forced to eliminate such activities as going to the beauty parlor and watching television. She claimed she hardly had time to prepare her clothing for work. The fact that her scrupulous attention to her husband's behavior was not appreciated by Mr Grasso troubled her. Nevertheless, she showed no inclination to reduce her involvement in the care. When laboratory results showed that Mr Grasso's condition was improving, the wife felt justified in her actions, and strengthened in her will to continue as home care supervisor.

The adjustments made in the Grasso home following hospitalization interfered with the normally close emotional ties the family enjoyed. Mr Grasso was "left out" of normal family affairs to a very considerable degree. There was an awkwardness to interpersonal relations. Home care roles were in the familiar role-differentiated style but they did not now facilitate companionship and communication. Mrs

Grasso had control, but Mr Grasso was isolated.

The following example of a not untypical evening in the home during the second stage of the home care illustrates the strain from the role adjustment. (It was constructed from my conversations with each family member):

> After dinner the books and papers relating to the store's operation were brought to the dining room and Anthony and Mrs Grasso began discussing the day's receipts, and planning for the upcoming Thanksgiving holiday. Decisions had to be made about how much new stock to order, how to display it, and whether or not to open early during the week of the holiday. Mr Grasso was sitting in the living room about twenty feet away and was turned toward the television. He could see and hear his wife and son through the wide passageway separating the two rooms. Mr Grasso said nothing, but later each person would report being highly conscious of his exclusion. Outwardly, all was calm. But this belied the tension each felt. While Mr Grasso seemed to ignore events in the next room, he was tuned in. When the others went to bed, Mr Grasso returned quietly to the dining room and examined the books and order forms. He was unaware that his son was watching him.

The Family Perception of the Medical Care System

As we have seen, a common problem which confronted everyone was uncertainty about the husband–patients' fitness to undertake activity at home. While husbands and wives were sometimes in disagreement over the extent to which activity posed a danger to health, all the spouses and children lived with an acute sense of doubt and fearful anticipation of potential illness reoccurrence. Yet, no one attempted to contact the family physician, either for reassurance when the newly homebound heart patient experienced symptoms of various kinds, including chest pain, or to try for an earlier appointment. Moreover, when people did see the family physician they did not generally seek his help in resolving the differences in interpretation of the regimen over which spouses often found themselves in conflict.

While this behavior may indicate that family members

were attempting to avoid facing up to their problems and so denied them, the fact that they were willing to express to this researcher not only their fears and conflicts, but also their need for medical system support, suggests alternative hypotheses. On the basis of remarks made to me by patients and other family members both prior to and after hospital discharge, there is evidence to claim that there was widespread misunderstanding of the role that the medical care system would play during the home-based recovery period, and much confusion over the role the family physician was to play. This seems to have contributed to confusion about the kind of services they could expect to receive from Medical Group, when they would receive them, and ultimately to a decline in confidence in the medical care system's professional expertise. Lack of sufficient knowledge of the role of the family physician, and of the system for continuity of inpatient and ambulatory services, rather than denial of problems, prevented the families from making more of a claim to the expertise and support of Medical Group. In view of the observations made at the start of the illness when delay in getting to Group Hospital resulted in several instances from lack of understanding of the procedures for utilizing emergency services, the finding of Roemer's (1972) study group seems to apply to Medical Group. They made the observation that organizational complexity of group practices can be a barrier to client utilization of services because people are unused to dealing with bureaucracies for their medical care.

As mentioned in Chapter 1, Medical Group's arrangement for coordinating in-patient and ambulatory patient care services was different from that provided by the traditional mode of health delivery under which health consumers pay a fee to a private practitioner for each service rendered. When clients of Medical Group enter Group Hospital, their family physicians do not provide direct patient care, as often occurs under the traditional form of medical care delivery in the United States. Rather, physicians on assignment to Group Hospital plan and carry out necessary diagnostic tests and therapeutic procedures. If the family physician so chooses, he can visit the patient in the hospital but cannot assume responsibility for the care. For example, the family physician will not order laboratory tests, or write orders for medication. The family physician does, however, resume patient care responsibilities once patients are discharged from the hospital.

Patients and family members attributed the absence of the family physician from the in-hospital phase of the care to limitations in his skill and knowledge. The family physician was perceived as less than adequate, by virtue of his training, to care for victims of heart attacks. In contrast, the physicians who provided care in the hospital were perceived as specially trained experts in heart disease. Patients and family members, therefore, expected to receive continuing medical care services after hospital discharge from other specialists, if not the same ones they had in the hospital. A short time after Mr Grasso had been home from the hospital, he reflected on the kind of continuing medical care his condition required. He said, "If I could have an examination by a good heart man, a good cardiologist, a good x-ray man, good blood people, good dietician . . . I'm sure it would head off any coming heart attack."

Several people mentioned at home that they wanted more than a periodic examination by a cardiologist; they wanted such specialists to be in full control of their care. Mr O'Shea responded to my question about when he was going to make an appointment with his family doctor this way:

Yes, my wife was down there and he [the family doctor] said he wanted to see me. She was a little confused about what went on. She told him I was supposed to see the doctor I had in the hospital. I'd like to get transferred to that doctor who is connected with Group Hospital. I think he's the resident in Internal Medicine . . . I imagine he is involved in the heart. So I think I'd be much better off if I could transfer to him . . . I guess the Internal Medicine group handles it after a heart attack, don't they? I'm not anxious to see that family doctor. I'd really like to see that [cardiologist]. (E.S.: What would you like to happen at that meeting with the cardiologist?) To find out how I'm coming along. If I can go back to this job I have.

Clients of Medical Group have the right to consultation by a specialist. The usual procedure is for the client's family physician to arrange for this when the person asks. However, Mr and Mrs Ambrosio expected that the specialist the family physician arranged for him to see would provide continuous care. His wife related that after they learned that this would not occur, and that the family physician was still the main source of care, they were both disappointed. She told me:

> On the way home I said "When does he want to see you again?" He said, "Oh, he won't have to see me anymore, just go back to [the family physician]." I said, "I think it could be a good idea if Dr Jones [the specialist] saw you all the time." He snapped at me and said, "Shut up." We were waiting so long to see Dr Jones and expected to be under his care . . . I was disappointed that Dr Jones didn't do more and then follow up. I felt he would be the internist's patient.

One of the claims made for the group practice mode of health delivery is that patient care can be made more rational and more efficient through the integration of research with service goals. Members of a larger group practice provide a defined population for basic sciences, epidemiologic, and social science research. Ideally, the finding of scientific studies contribute to effective coordination of medical care services.

At the time the eight men in my study were patients, Medical Group was involved in a study to learn the long term physiological effects of myocardial infarction. Either just before or after they were discharged from Group Hospital, each of the men was asked to participate in this project. All but one patient and spouse failed to distinguish this research project from medical care. In other words, most people believed that this was Medical Group's procedure for providing them with the expert care they believed they needed. Since they were told they would be contacted for testing within a short period, some people may have felt that there was no need to request a specialist consultation from the family physician. It appears that patients benefited from participating in this research activity of Medical Group because test results were supposed to be passed on to the family physician. However, a potential disadvantage for the system and the patient was that in misunderstanding the purpose of the research project, patients may have failed to utilize medical care services which they felt they needed, and to which they were entitled. For example, had they known that the testing to which they were invited was primarily for research purposes, more patients may have asked to be seen by specialists, and they may have requested this soon after hospital discharge. Several persons I spoke with after their testing said that it was less helpful to them than they had expected because "it's only research."

Had patients and family members known earlier that the major responsibility for their care rested with the family physician, they might have utilized him more effectively. Believing that a physician more expert in matters directly pertaining to their needs would soon be involved in their care, people may have had reservations in accepting the advice of the family doctor, and postponed asking many questions. They may have preferred to wait for the chance to talk with "the expert." Based on what patients and their spouses told me of what transpired during their visits to the family physician, they asked few questions of the doctors and reported having as many doubts about their condition and what to do about it after the meeting with the family physician as they had before they went.

On the other hand, it is possible to argue that by the time the patient was discharged from the hospital his expectation that he needed a higher degree of expert help than his family physician could provide was already firmly established. By that time he may already have determined that he neither needed nor wanted the assistance of the family physician for this health problem. In a very real sense the organization of Medical Group's health care delivery system may have created needs and expectations among the patients and their spouses which the system never intended, and therefore, could not subsequently meet.

To review, at the start of home care, each family faced hard problems. The most worrisome arose from lack of confidence that the home environment could protect the recovering heart attack victim from relapse. Without the direct supervision of medical experts, wives, children, and patient–husbands were afraid to make independent judgements to interpret the medical care regimen. Instead they took what was felt to be the safest course, i.e., having the patient adopt a routine modeled on the Intensive Care Unit. As difficult as this period – The Extension of Hospitalization – was, the source of family problems were seen by the members to be from the outside. The illness was conceived as an external threat and the members joined forces to protect themselves from its effects. Consequently, interpersonal family relationships were generally harmonious. Working together seemed to bring a measure of well-being to families under the threat of crisis.

The nature of the problems families faced changed in a qualitative way, however, once the patient–husbands decided to become more active. Since their decisions were based on definitions of the recovery process which were not shared by their spouses, the tendency was for wives to oppose the actions of the husbands. Now family members blamed each other for thwarting the chances for recovery. Family problems centered on conflict between members.

As we saw in Chapters 2 and 3, discrepencies in families in understanding the nature of the threat of illness and the requirements of the recovery process originated during hospitalization. The consequences of this lack of consensus, however, only surfaced a week or two after hospital discharge. Because there were no organized mechanisms at Group Hospital to allow definitions of the situation to emerge, the families were not able to work through their differences at a time when professional social service or psychiatric personnel could have helped. Instead family members had to cope alone in a situation already tense and worrisome. The fact that lack of coordination in the hospital between patient and family experiences produced problems when the patient arrived home had no way of being fed back to the hospital staff for system correction. Since a large part of the social and psychiatric services available to patients and their families are allocated on the basis of referrals made by hospital medical and nursing staff, one can see how many families that could profit from professional counseling go undetected and unserved.

We saw from the analysis made in this chapter that strategies for managing the home care reflected the organization of the family. Whether the family's structure and value climate would have played such an important role in organizing the home care had the medical care system played a more active role is hard to assess.

People in divergent family systems were the first to disengage from acute care roles which were adopted at the start of homecoming. As a result, patients in these families began the process of resuming pre-illness roles earlier than their counterparts in the two other types of family. Their early mobilization was aided by the general feeling of discomfort in their families with the type of interaction fostered by a patient–nurse surrogate relationship. Segregating members into highly reciprocal interdependent roles was antithetical with the arrangements that were valued and practised prior to the onset of the illness. With an aim toward avoiding conflict which had surfaced when wives tried to play controlling nurse–surrogate roles to husbands' passive patient roles, the couples opted for a home care division of labor that allowed each partner to participate. Their strategy for dealing with home care management was basically a way of balancing the requirement of the recovery with the demands of family norms and mores.

People in convergent and discordant family systems remained in patient and nurse–surrogate roles for a longer period and the men had fewer opportunities to test their abilities to resume activity. We saw that for couples that had been in conflict prior to the illness over role expectations and performances, the reorganized home care role arrangement brought a significant degree of harmony to marital relationships. There was social gain from the illness in these families.

The Grassos, a convergent family, experienced considerable strain in relationships. Home care roles were maintained by coercive efforts of wife and son against a patient, who, while accepting the principle of a role differentiated division of labor, had considerable difficulty accepting the limitations the sick role posed to his sense of self. The son, too, was emotionally shaken by the role he felt obliged to play in controlling his father's behavior. The wife, deeply committed to maintaining the form if not the substance of the conjugal pattern, perceived herself as having no choice but to hold tightly the reins of home care management. Motivated by her felt obligation to guide her husband safely to recovery, and by her concern for stabilizing valued family patterns, she accepted short term social and emotional costs for long term benefits.

Given a context for rehabilitation in which family structure and culture influences how people behave after hospital discharge, it is significant that the medical care system left rehabilitation decision making so exclusively in the realm of the family of the patient.

[1] This diagram appears by kind permission of the Family Service Association of America, publishers of *Social Casework*. It originally appeared in Reuben Hill's article, 'Generic Features of Families under Stress', *Social Casework*, February–March 1958.

6

Normalization: The Costs of Reentering Normal Social Roles

Several authors (Bermann 1973, Farber 1964, Jackson 1956) have taken up the theme first suggested by Reuben Hill (1958) that the family's response to crisis is like a ride on a roller-coaster. What seems to be a typical experience is that no sooner has a family managed to cope with one set of problems when it is suddenly beset with new, unanticipated difficulties: uncertainties in anticipating the pace of recovery, discrepancies between peoples' definitions of what is expected of the disease, and sudden shifts in the ill person's condition. Strauss (1975:47) explains that at each step in the patient's career,

> the ill person must reassess where he is and therefore what social arrangements are necessary in order to manage his symptoms, social relations, daily life, and preparations for his life in the foreseeable future . . . In a genuine sense, any chronically ill person who phases drastically down, or up for that matter, becomes a new person in the house.

As we look at what our subjects have so far experienced, the roller-coaster analogy seems to fit. The first one and a half to two months of home based recovery have brought both joys and sorrows, with some people experiencing more of one than the other. But what is most striking is the volatile nature of the situation, and, inspite of attempts within most groups to structure modes of adaptation, its unpredictability. For even as the aforementioned responses to the strains of home care were being fashioned, the situation changed.

Recall that for the first six to eight weeks at home the men had been either doing very little (Messrs Warren, Shea, Goldberg) or were following a schedule which bore little resemblance to their former lifestyles (Messrs Ambrosio, Asti, Grasso, and Stein); only Mr Polski took a fast track toward normalizing his life. Many of the problems being grappled with involved the location of a set of activities that the patients found meaningful and that satisfied the collective definition of what was permissable and appropriate medically. Fairly large arguments could occur over how many blocks the patient should walk, or whether lifting the garbage can was too strenuous an activity? Fashioning a workable compromise between conflicting points of view on these matters was no small achievement as our earlier examples show.

Sometime around the third month of home care, a change occurred in most of the homes which brought about a crisis atmosphere once again. It may have been coming on gradually, imperceptibly, but it seemed that most men, following a strong inner need, suddenly decided to move their activities into the mainstream of what for them was normal. In a sudden rush, they quickened their pace and attempted to regain those activities that formerly were theirs and that either had been assumed by others or abandoned since their heart attack.

The men explained their behavior in terms of urgency, as if there were a pressing need which could wait no longer for their attention. And they seemed willing to accept as consequences increased fatigue, discomfort, and anxiety.

Mr Polski used his son's impending return from military service as the reason for increasing his efforts to finish constructing his country home. He claimed that because he had promised to give his son this house, he had to have it ready for him and could not stop work, even if pain or fatigue increased as a consequence. Mr Asti focused on an upcoming trip to Florida as he took on the heaviest activities since his heart attack. He told me:

> See, one of the things I did do in the last couple of weeks I was doubtful about doing. I was afraid to do it, but I went ahead anyway. I changed the plugs in the car . . . tuned the car up. I was doubtful whether I should do it or not, but I went ahead and did it anyhow . . . I was concerned about

doing it. I felt maybe I was doing the wrong thing . . . even though the doctor had said he didn't want me to drive to Florida. My wife would drive, my brother-in-law would drive. I wanted to make sure nothing went wrong with the car . . . As it turned out, we decided to fly down. If I had known that I wouldn't have done it.

Concurrent with this development was the emergence of a theme in the interviews which has been referred to in other studies as the fear of premature social aging (Singer 1974). In this context, the men seemed to fear that continuing to be relatively inactive, remaining within the confines of the sick role, could conceivably lead to permanent disability.

The sense of urgency may have had less to do with specific tasks than with time itself, which appeared to be running out. Mr Polski remarked,

Maybe I'm harming myself by not sitting down in a rocking chair like they want me to. I'll be 65 next week [long pause]. If I sit down I'm not going to get any younger, and if I sit down for a month I'm going to be that much older, and I won't want to get up anymore and do these things. While I still have the urge and ambition to do it, I want to do these things.

Mr Grasso echoed this theme:

I cannot say, "OK, I'll sit in the easy chair and you take care of me." It might make her very happy if I say I'm not going to go to work anymore, I'm going to put on my slippers, I won't smoke anymore, I'll put on an old sweater and watch TV. I won't lift a thing the rest of my life. She might be happy. But I'll be miserable. And I'm selfish at least that much, to say I don't want to be that kind of miserable to make people happy . . . So I've got to contribute something, so I'm going to go out and do some work.

These sentiments were present in the earlier stages of the rehabilitative process, but they were submerged by the overriding concern with the possibility of reinjury. Then, the men thought, "I should be grateful I'm still around, period!"

Now the fear was not so much with whether recovery would be achieved, but would it be achieved *in time*. Months after returning home from the hospital, the timetable for resuming a full measure of normality was still vaguely open ended.

The full expression of this concern was articulated by Mr Ambrosio who perhaps was speaking for many who move from middle to old age only to be saddled with the oppression of illness.

It's a difficult thing to try to readjust . . . trying to come back to a new type of living, thinking, acting. When you've been doing certain things for a given period and just to sit down, it's the toughest thing in the world . . . Sometimes time *never* moves. At other times, when you get older, there is only twenty hours in a day. There is never enough time. But to a young kid going to school the clock never moves . . . But as you get older there are so many things to get done and you have such a limited time to do it . . . By the grace of God we're here. You could be sitting here and "Bam," you're in never, never, land. If you had time you'd say: "Gee, I wish I could have done this or that." But you never can wish.

In contrast with his own concern with the passage of time, Mr Ambrosio perceived his physician as having a more sanguine attitude. An example of this contrast in time perspectives occurred when Mr Ambrosio asked for permission to resume driving. The doctor was reported to have said, "Take it easy. Do you have to go anywhere? Do you have to go to work? No. So why worry about it?" Mr Ambrosio grew increasingly worried. He could not target a time when he would take up, once again, those activities which gave meaning to his existence. He worried that he would, through inactivity, lose the vitality he valued so highly.

For Messrs Ambrosio, Grasso, Polski, Asti, and Stein, visiting the physician had become frustrating. While Mr Asti continued to look forward to these visits, he left them not knowing exactly what he should be doing. He could not grasp the essence of "go at your own pace." Mr Polski tried to elicit from his physician a way to regain his ebbing strength. He asked for "pep pills", inquired about the possibility of heart surgery to correct his anatomical anomaly, and finally argued to increase the nitroglycerine prescription so he could at least withstand the pain that accompanied his daily labors. Mr Ambrosio expressed his feelings this way, "I'm tired of hearing 'Don't do this, don't do that.' I want to know what I can do!"

Unable to elicit from their physicians a means of achieving entry into a state of normality, the men began to chart their own course. With no apologies, Mr Polski refused to be guided by less than his own inclinations and struggled to recapture his former lifestyle. Mr Ambrosio attempted to redefine his health problem. He explained his position this way.

> The doctor said... "When you start to get tired, when you get a shortage of breath, stop." I said, "Can I tell you something? Since the day I came out of the hospital... I have not had any pains or aches. I get no shortness of breath." And, of course, as I said many times [but not to me or his wife until this point] I still believe that it was the diabetes and not my heart per se... I don't have these symptoms, I know there was something wrong, but to what degree? It might have been minimal compared with what these other fellows had [who were in the hospital with him]. (E.S.: Did you mention this opinion of yours to either doctor?) Well, I talked to them, but you know, they look at you with a cork screw eye: Who the hell are you to tell us ... So they sort of discounted it. He said, "No, you had a definite coronary." They always associate the diabetes as secondary to the coronary. In my opinion, it is the diabetes and then the coronary.

Mr Grasso also argued that the main problem now was diabetes: "I worry more about the diabetes, because I can't control the heart, but I can control the sugar. Whatever has gotten to it, I can't do anything about it."

These changes in attitude and in behavior were followed by the re-emergence of conflict in the families involved. The wives responded with a combination of fear and anger and the children seemed thrown in confusion.

The intensity of the ensuing struggle was greater by far

than it had been previously. No period in the illness crisis was as conflict ridden for the families than the one that followed the onset of husband–patients' normalization activities. No period brought as much emotional hurt to the members or so disturbed family solidarity.

It was generally agreed that the conflict over normalization was equal to, and in some cases, surpassed what the family had experienced in its history. As a consequence of the hostilities, two wives threatened to separate from their husbands. Moreover, three wives reported their own health was adversely affected: Mrs Ambrosio had her first attack of osteoarthritis since before the heart attack; Mrs Stein, who herself suffered from angina pectoris, had to increase her dosage of nitroglycerine; Mrs Polski went to the doctor complaining of unexplained weight loss and dizzy spells.

In contrast, life in the O'Shea, Goldberg, and Warren families, where the men continued to behave very cautiously and inactively, was not so troubled. These men accepted the prospect of long term disability. Accepting disability seemed to shield against family conflict.

Interestingly, Mr O'Shea also faced a problem with his physician. However, what Mr O'Shea wished to obtain from his physician was a sanction not to return to work, but to go into semi-retirement.

In addition to family fighting over what the regimen allowed and did not allow the men to do, the tension the men felt because of their own uncertainty over their activities contributed to the climate of unhappiness. Mr Asti found one "important task" to do after another. Each he approached warily, even at times fearfully, but with determination. For example, I asked him, "You said you felt tired, does that mean you had pain?" Mr Asti replied, "No, but I was under tension. I didn't know if it was going to be harmful or not. It wasn't much as far as physical exertion is concerned . . . I was just worried about the after effects, would they cause me pain or harmful affects afterward?" The tension that he experienced seemed to be directly related to the changes that occurred in his behavior toward others in the home. Rose, his daughter, summed up his behavior as "nasty." He became uncharacteristically critical of others, and then seemed to withdraw by not talking to anyone. This behavior caused his wife to become angry at him and there was bitterness and loud shouting in the home. Activities he was engaging in at this time were substantial ones: cementing the patio, shoveling snow. He claimed that he had to do these things when his wife objected or else "the whole patio will get ruined;" or "someone will slip." Rose herself vascillated between arguing with her mother to stop "nagging" him, getting angry with her father over his "nastiness," and withdrawing completely and spending time away from home.

As Mr Polski pushed to finish building his home, his chest pains increased to the point where he was taking over ten nitroglycerine pills a day. He said he took his frustrations out on his wife. "I get aggravated and I do take it out on my wife . . . It is only when I'm working, doing something and I'm bothered. It is bothering me to get these pains. It is such a simple thing and I can't do it anymore." His wife who earlier had seemed satisfied with the recovery process, greeted me one morning in the following manner: ES: [as I arrived] "How are things?" Mrs Polski: [shaking her head and laughing sorrowfully] "He hasn't been feeling too good. He has been so cranky. I feel sorry for him. But what can I do? He yells all the time" [she begins crying].

Another wife, Mrs Ambrosio, told me at the time when her husband started becoming more active: "I think I am really getting on his nerves the last few days. Really, it has not been too good." (ES: Why is that, do you think?) "He feels that I am telling him too many things. He is really getting uptight." She went on to describe a fight they recently had in which "he really blew his top" and said things to her which upset her greatly.

A difficulty all these families faced was a lack of being able to predict what the patient–husband would do next, and when hostilities would emerge. The patients themselves were not sure what they should do or could do, and how they would feel afterward. They advanced toward normalization filled with uncertainty. They seemed often to have no systematic plan of recovering past activities and often made spur-of-the-moment decisions. For the wives this meant that they could not organize their time, as some of them had before, to be present to counsel and help when their husbands were likely to be active. Some reported that they went out only to find that the men had done some large task. Mrs Ambrosio, for example, found that her husband plastered the ceiling one afternoon in her absence. This precipitated conflict. She resolved to stay home as much as she possibly could.

This normalization period was characterized by lack of trust. People could not count on each other to behave in accordance with one set of norms. Shocks became commonplace. Mrs Stein said: "I never know what kind of a mood he is going to be in when I get home." Patients, on the other hand, accused their wives of blaming them without cause, and treating them like children.

Although families were confronted with the same problem, the struggle to deal with it took different forms. Again, family structure and value climate seemed to predict the mode of problem solving that followed.

Normalization in Divergent Families

The tendency for the husbands increasingly to take on tasks within the home without regard for either wifely or medical advice made it exceedingly difficult for the wives to remain involved in the recovery process without directly opposing this behavior. They still felt an obligation to help prevent the reoccurrence of illness, and perceived their husbands' present behavior to be dangerous. When they did try to intervene, however, the result was often conflict.

Since a part of the wife's strategy included staying aware of her husband's behavior in order to try to persuade against over-activity, the times when she felt constrained to argue with him increased steadily. In addition, the higher level of activity made wives and children highly sensitive to any symptoms the men exhibited. In fact, Mr Stein had severe chest pain and required rehospitalization. Tests revealed that blood clots had formed in his legs presenting the danger that one would eventually lodge in the heart. Mr Polski's chest pain increased steadily and he took large amounts of nitroglycerine to control the pain while he worked. Mr Asti felt "burning" in the chest. Whether these symptoms were brought on by the activity or by anxiety is not entirely clear. The wives struggled briefly against the activities of their husbands. For a time the divergent homes were conflict ridden. Soon, however, the wives in these homes disengaged once again from efforts to control their spouses' behavior. Up until the time this study ended, a process of withdrawal from their role in the recovery process took place.

The withdrawal of the wives was begun by redefining the situation in two ways: first, by decreasing their opportunities for observing "deviant" behavior; second, by transferring responsibility to the men themselves for interpreting and implementing the recovery process.

It was during the period when the men were moving toward normalizing their lives that their wives took important steps to resume their own pre-illness lifestyles. Consequently, they spent more time outside the home, and refocused their attention when in the home. For example, Mrs Asti resumed her recreational activities which included playing cards at friends' homes, and going alone or with friends to the bingo parlor. She also began special house-cleaning projects which absorbed several daytime hours. Mrs Polski also made arrangements for visiting and shopping trips with her friends. Steadily her own interests took her from where she would be absorbed with what her husband was doing. I asked her if she was still involved with trying to limit her husband's activities. She replied: "I ask, but I can't wait around all day." Mrs Stein told me she tried to act like "like everything was OK". She did this by trying to attend to her sewing and reading when she came home from work, and by not insisting, as she had done earlier, on serving her husband dinner.

In accounting for their change in approach, wives like Mrs Asti shrugged: "I don't know; I guess if he feels like doing it it's alright . . . he knows what to do, he doesn't need to be told." Mrs Polski put it more bluntly, "He doesn't need to be told; he knows when he doesn't stop he has pains. He's a big boy now."

Conflict could be reduced but not eradicated entirely. Inner tension still produced hostile words and deeds. But, by all accounts, wives of men who were struggling to shed the sick role attempted not to fight fire with fire. Mrs Stein gives an example.

> He gets very upset with me. (ES: Is that different than before?) Yes, I talk loud. I cannot modulate my tone. I happen to be the type of woman who has a loud voice. I'm trying very, very hard to speak softly. Lots of times when we are talking he tells me, "What are you hollering for? I cannot even talk without you hollering." I said, "I'm not." He said, "Oh yes you are." So there is that conflict that I never had with him before. He knows my tone of voice . . . (ES: When he says things like that how do you respond?) I tell him I'm sorry. That ends it then and there. I'm sorry.

Mrs Polski said that she always knew when her husband was in pain because he was "cranky and irritable." She said that his behavior prevented her from talking much to him: "I'll say: 'Let it go. You did enough for today.' He gets mad. I don't say anything. I walk away. I ease my conscience by telling him to take it easy, then it is up to him . . . When he hollers I shut up. It would only drag it out."

As we have been attempting to show, these adaptations are understandable in the light of the climate of values in divergent families: individual preferences predominate. Moreover, it was typical to respond to problems by decreasing interactive and increasing social distance.

There is another aspect that comes into play, however. Transferring responsibility to the men, extricated the wives from potential blame should any relapse occur. Without the means of controlling the situation, they had little to gain by continuing the fray.

Individual Differences in Divergent Family Behavior During the Normalizing Phase

Transferring responsibility to the husband while reengaging formerly satisfying life patterns was not accomplished with the same amount of ease in each family. Individual differences in how families stabilized their behavior patterns seem related to the following sets of circumstances:

1 *If the man's health improved and did not show signs of deteriorating under his lifestyle, and his wife was successful at normalizing her own social life, the family was able to function smoothly. The crisis appeared to be over.* (The Astis)

2 *If the man's health deteriorated under his lifestyle, yet the wife was successful at normalizing her own social life, interpersonal conflict, while present, was kept within tolerable limits.* (The Polskis)

3 *If the man's health deteriorated, and the wife was unsuccessful at normalizing her own social life, family life was severely disorganized. The family crisis deepened.* (The Steins)

Emerging From Crisis – The Asti Family

Like the other families where the men were determined to leave the sick role behind, the Asti's lived through a very difficult, conflict-ridden period. Neither spouse was confident in returning to normal, pre-illness patterns. Mr Asti approached each new activity with a dread of what the consequences would be. Feeling discomfort in his chest did not restrain him from doing more, it just made him more anxious. To his wife, he still appeared unwell. She said he was pale, and his eyes didn't look clear. Her memory of friends and relatives who had died from heart attacks was a constant reminder of the need for her husband to be cautious.

Mrs Asti tried to compensate for reducing her own involvement in her husband's care. She tried to induce her married daughter to substitute for her, and she continued to call upon relatives to volunteer their help in chores. Neither made much of an impact on his pace. Mr Asti was described as continually highly strung and argumentative. With conflict ever ready to emerge.

Mrs Asti refocused her attention on her own activities and she was instrumental in keeping the members of the nuclear family from confrontations. She urged her children not to respond when their father seemed to provoke arguments with them. What she in effect told them was: listen, and then ignore him. He had become uncharacteristically invasive of his children's privacy and critical of their behavior at home. He yelled at Rose for not cleaning her room, and for not responding quickly enough to suit him when he asked her something. Mrs Asti also urged her husband not to pay attention to what the children were doing. In effect, she was invoking a normal response.

The children, who were accustomed to spending a good deal of time away from home, and when at home, to be by themselves, increased their separateness even more. John, it was reported, was not around as much as he usually was. Moreover, he seemed to avoid occasions of friction with his father by refraining from requesting favors such as borrowing the car. I was told that prior to the illness, refusal to let John borrow the car led, occasionally, to arguments with Mr Asti. Rose's strategy was to spend more time at the home of her boyfriend, or in her own room. She also assiduously avoided answering her father back. There was also a noticeable decrease in interaction between Mrs Asti and her daughter Rose.

Lack of intrafamily interaction and withdrawal of the members into their own personal worlds did reduce the occasions for conflict without creating a serious problem in terms of feelings of mutual hostility or estrangement. Family members told me they believed this was the "best way" to protect themselves from conflict and defined the withdrawal and avoidance as mutually beneficial.

No one seemed to blame Mr Asti for his bad moods. Mr Asti's wife and children spoke of the reasons he had for feeling and acting irritably. They blamed the situation and felt these moods would pass. In the meantime they would continue to give him a wide berth.

Mrs Asti left her husband to himself and went about her own business in and out of the house. Her role in the care narrowed to control over the diet. She continued making all his low sodium, low fat meals. She seemed to build up this role and defined her responsibilities almost totally in terms of trying to effect a weight loss in her husband.

Conditions in the family changed dramatically following an examination of Mr Asti by a physician affiliated with his union. Mr Asti's union required its sick members to consult with one of its own physicians for clearance either for return to work or for continuance of sick leave benefits.

Two factors made this a "landmark" experience for Mr Asti. He said the doctor was an "internist," someone who he believed had special training in the area of the heart. As such, his credibility with Mr Asti was considerably higher than the family doctor's.

This physician's approach seemed particularly suited to Mr Asti's needs. He reviewed his activities and then told Mr Asti to *do more* than he was already doing. "He took the fear of doing too much away from me," Mr Asti reported. The way that Mr Asti described their meeting, the doctor presented an active, authoritative image which was convincing. The doctor discounted Mr Asti's fear about the "burning sensation" in his chest. His own family doctor had told him not to worry about this in the past. Yet, for over a month in every contact I had with Mr Asti, he expressed concern about it, and anxiety over his schedule of activities.

When I observed the change in Mr Asti's morale subsequent to this examination, I realized how deep had been his worry. The internist said not to worry and he seemed to believe him. Mr and Mrs Asti took a week's vacation to Florida and reported it was a happy time. For the first time Mr Asti was able to reduce his weight, which the couple thought was remarkable since in Florida the relatives they were visiting prepared special Italian style meals, rich in sauce and pasta. Somehow, as his morale went up, his weight went down.

The family came together again – within their normal boundaries. Mrs Asti even asked her husband to help her with some chores around the house. Mr Asti was looking forward to returning to work in a few weeks. Rose said that she went out now when she wanted to, and since her father was no longer "nasty" she felt no need to stay away from home longer than she wanted to. There was no evidence that the conflict the family had recently experienced had left any bitter aftermath. Indeed, the value of their problem solving techniques seemed to have been confirmed in their eyes.

Looking forward toward the future, Mr Asti said he would "slow down" a little. For example, he planned to save his heavy household chores for weekends rather than starting them after work. But, he indicated that life for him and his family would go on as normal.

Conflict Tolerance – The Polskis

During the second stage of the home care, the relationship between Mr and Mrs Polski had been amicable. Both were optimistic about his health, and the couple was able to play their respective roles of patient and nurse with flexibility. The climate in the home was shattered by a serious intensification of symptoms of illness after Mr Polski increased his activities. Rather than reduce the extent of work in building the house, Mr Polski increased his intake of nitroglycerine, which sometimes went as high as over twenty pills a day. As soon as the pain subsided, he went back to work.

As the other wives had attempted to do, Mrs Polski tried to stop him from working. Her arguments and direct efforts to intervene by helping him get done faster so he could rest were almost complete failures. Both spouses were candid about the extent to which they were drawn into conflict over this issue. Both realized that he would not reduce his activities, and planned to increase them. Even when she said she withdrew from interfering with her husband and only offered to help him, she claimed, and he agreed, that hostilities continued to beset them. "I want to do as much as I can for him, but he never talks nice to me. He is always yelling. I can't seem to please him." Then she reasoned: "It's not going to stop. I have to get used to it. One of us has to give."

Mrs Polski was the one who gave in. First, she fled at the first sign of conflict. She did not completely stop expressing her opinion of the "correct" way of recuperating. But when her husband responded in anger, she was silent. She told me she refused to respond once he became angry, but walked away, leaving him alone. There were certain elements of passive–aggression in this since she said Mr Polski would have welcomed an argument to release his own tensions. She realized that walking away sometimes made her husband angrier. But Mrs Polski claimed that she could not bear the constant arguing. She herself paid a price. She told me, "It's hard to hold it all inside."

It was at this point that Mrs Polski returned to a very important part of her life – visiting her friends in the city. Since the start of the illness, she had not taken her usual long visits to the city. During the optimistic and amicable part of the home care, she claimed she had an obligation to stay with her husband. She explained then: "I'd feel terrible if something happened when I was away." Making the decision to leave her husband for the several days these trips lasted took into consideration her feeling that: "There is nothing I can do here." She told me that her husband was aware of the risks he was taking and was not uninformed of the fact that his family doctor had recommended that he do less, especially in light of the chronic pain. "He doesn't need anyone to tell him," she said, "he knows when he gets pain he should stop."

Going into the city was a great lift to her morale, "Thank God for my friends," she exclaimed. She did not completely stop responding to his pain or suggesting at times he should do less. But she was able to choose the occasions to do this, and being away more they fought less, and she seemed to be able to maintain a satisfying life. When we spoke of her experiences with her husband, she showed her disappointment at his declining health and she cried over how she felt about the conflict. But when she recalled the typical events of her day, she perked up and seemed for a while to forget the bad times in the home as she told me of the good times outside, in the country and the city.

While Mrs Polski resumed her life with her friends, Mr Polski worked to finish the basement of the home in the country. He worked as long and as hard as his pain and fatigue would allow. With the help of nitroglycerine, he continued heavy construction work until his death from a sudden heart attack, about five months after first entering the hospital.

Mr Polski was aware that his doctor wanted him to cut down, not increase his activities. This was not acceptable to him. He said he would prefer death over "living as an invalid." He perceived no middle ground between full activity and invalidism.

Mr Polski was not able to accept a modified lifestyle even though when he rested he was relatively free of physical discomfort. At the height of these troubles he traded in his automobile for a small truck so he could haul even more material for his projects. Once he told me that for him life without work was not worth living. He worked until he died.

Continuing Deterioration – The Steins

As mentioned, Mr Stein was readmitted to the hospital because of a problem of blood clotting. When he returned home the second time, Mrs Stein took an approach toward her role in his case that was decidedly different from the one she took the first time. She did not stay home from work as she had before and commented that then "I was overly protective . . . he was getting annoyed with me . . . if he dropped anything I went to pick it up. I have a bad back so I have to watch how I bend. That, I know, was annoying him."

Nevertheless, when the couple was together, it was apparent that there was much tension in their relationship. As we sat together over coffee, they seemed unsure of what to say to each other and how to say it. Deciding who would serve coffee, for example, resulted in a brief but sharp exchange between them. When Mr Stein left the room for a moment, his wife just lowered her eyes and shook her head. She often complained, "I never had this with him before."

Mrs Stein feared that his health was steadily deteriorating, and believed his actions contributed. Sometimes she told me she just had to express her concern and her anger. For example, Mr Stein was smoking two packs of cigarettes a day, driving the car, and making repairs in the house which involved climbing and lifting. Arguing with him to cease these activities was to no avail. The fact that she could have so little impact on his behavior was a source of continuous personal grief because in her view, he needed someone to guide his recovery. She expressed her problem to me this way:

I'm very short tempered with him which is very bad I know . . . I have very, very guilty complexes – the fact that I have to leave him alone. The fact that I tried to interest him in something and it didn't work. The fact that he climbed up and changed the light bothered me. He did that when I wasn't here. He stood on that chair. Now, God forbid, had he fallen off or something, that bothers me. A lot of things are bothering me.

Ordinarily, she did not want to inquire about the outcome of various tests he took to determine the extent of his blood clotting problem. It was inevitable that she would learn, however. When she did and the news was bad, she could not control the emotion she felt. Sometimes she learned new dimensions of the illness when her husband told me about them. On one occasion he told me, in her presence, some particularly disappointing news. The lab result indicated that a danger point had been reached. To control the clotting he was required for the next few days to take such a high dosage of medication that there was a danger he would suffer internal bleeding. When Mrs Stein heard this, she bolted upright in the chair and a look of worried concern covered her face. A few moments later, she left the room and did not return. Mr Stein then observed that his wife was quite unable to bear up under such news and that he had to censor the statements he made to her about his health.

Managing the bad news was a source of strain to both persons. His knowledge that she could not tolerate it led him to mask it. When it was revealed, it came to Mrs Stein as a shock. Mr Stein indicated he felt under-supported. He asked: "What would happen if I have an emergency at home? Who would be able to take charge?"

Other wives we saw were able to reactivate their outside social groups and interests and were thereby somewhat shielded from trouble inside the home. Mrs Stein had few interests which took her out of the home. She still went to work, but at home could not engage easily in the activities that normally brought her satisfaction. She said that after work:

There are times when I don't want to see anybody, hear voices. I don't even want to pick up a phone. I'm with people five days a week, eight hours a day. All I do is talk, talk, talk. There are times on the weekends I don't want to see or hear anybody. I want to come in, close the door and just forget. Now, it's different. Now he seems to get tense as the evening wears on. If I ask him something, he'll just give me a dirty look.

It seemed that a major source of strain was the fact that neither person could give to the other the support that was desired. Mr Stein felt his wife was not competent to collaborate with him on ways of managing his illness. She seemed to him to lack knowledge and skill to prepare his diet properly. She also seemed to him to be uninformed about the regimen. She also did not support his decision to do as much as possible in spite of symptoms. Her arguments against his activities were perceived as another burden he had to cope with. Mrs Stein felt she could not win the concessions from her husband that would have given her a feeling of constructive involvement in his care. When she tried to rekindle the affection that she had known before the illness, she claimed he refused to reciprocate. Finally, she could not withdraw to the comfort of her separate lifestyle. Mrs Stein suffered a heart attack and died several months after my last conversation with her.

Normalization in Convergent and Discordant Families

Mr Grasso and Mr Ambrosio first emerged from a sedentary, patient-oriented mode of behavior to an active, task-oriented one at times when they were least likely to be observed by their wives. They began attempting arduous activities, and returned to premorbid habits like smoking, drinking coffee, doing chores secretly. This stands in contrast to the openness with which other men behaved.

When Mrs Grasso and Mrs Ambrosio learned that their husbands were acting one way in their presence and another when they were alone, it created a serious practical problem. The two wives had to re-evaluate their strategies for managing family affairs and maintaining control of the recovery process. The pattern which they had evolved during the second stage of home care seemed less than adequate now. The wives immediately rescheduled their time so that they could more effectively observe and limit their husbands' behavior. For example, when I asked Mrs Ambrosio about her activities outside of the home, like shopping, visiting friends, and so on, she replied: "It doesn't work out. When I come home I find that he has been doing something that he is not supposed to do, like plastering. He did the porch ceiling."

Mrs Grasso, who was employed four days a week made it a practice of stopping by the family store on her way home to be certain that her husband was not lifting heavy objects, and was sitting as often as he could. She also received information from a clerk who worked in the store.

This strategy of trying to induce conformity by observation of the husbands not only complicated the womens' daily routines, but also led to a climate of *distrust* in the homes. The men reported that they resented the extensive questioning they were subject to when the wives came home. At the same time, they felt the need to expand their activities. Mr Ambrosio told me: "I've got to fix a fixture over there in the hall, the light went out... That means getting a ladder out in the garage. Now I know that my wife is not going to let me get the ladder, so I may not be able to do it until she is not around." Mr Grasso's son, Anthony, told me that he noticed that his father was taking precautions, like keeping the front door locked so he would have time to dispose of evidence of smoking or working.

On the other hand, the two men argued that their wives were themselves manipulative. For example, Mr Ambrosio believed that his wife influenced the doctor to postpone certain activities:

E.S.:   Did the doctor give you a date for driving?
Mr Ambrosio: He didn't give me anything.
E.S.:   I thought it was going to be mid-April.
Mr Ambrosio: I have a sneaky feeling my wife is going to put that off no matter how well I plead my case ... When I get through with him, fine, everything is O.K.
E.S.:   Then she will go in?
Mr Ambrosio: He will say to her "Do you have any questions?" [she speaks to the doctor privately]. Then she comes out smiling. I say "What happened?" "Oh, fine." Then we get home and for a day or so she won't let on what happened.

The response of these wives in this situation contains no suggestion of voluntary withdrawal from their former positions. On the contrary, they increased their resolve to remain in control even in the face of heightening inter- and intrapersonal tension.

It is difficult to overlook the fact that for their wives normalization would bring a return of certain pre-morbid patterns which they objected to and which had been a serious source of concern to them prior to the illness. Specifically, Mr and Mrs Ambrosio had been in serious disagreement over how the household division of labor ought to be arranged; the Grassos were divided in their opinions concerning the work role of Mr Grasso. It is clear that the path the wives were following and were urging their husbands to follow would have resolved these issues – in the wives' favor. In other words, the conflict between the spouses which focused specifically on the definition of the illness and on interpretations of the medical regimen had implications of a wider sort. Control over the organization of the family was at stake. The outcome of patient rehabilitation would affect the nature of the marital dyad. The nurse role gave the wife more power and influence over her husband's behavior than she had previously. This power could be used to alter existing marital patterns to her greater satisfaction. If the man returned to a full normalization, she would lose this leverage.

Emerging from Crisis Through Disability – The Grasso Family

Events had created a house divided. In their struggle to overcome the illness, the members lost sense of the common goal. Each fought a separate battle. Mrs Grasso fought for a future in which her husband's health would be preserved through his adherence to a regimen of restricted activity, rest, no smoking, and especially a job that made limited demands on his energy. Mr Grasso fought to preserve his sense of self worth which he defined by his ability to be a successful businessman. The son, Anthony, struggled with his allegiance. He groped for a middle ground between his parents' positions.

The problems laid heavily on each. Mrs Grasso was worn out, both physically and emotionally. The long silences were harder for her to cope with than the bitter arguments and recriminations. She said she sometimes tried to reduce her role and not fight with him about his activities around the house, and in the store, but she could not remain silent for long. She said it caused constant fighting but she had to "nag him." Her resolve to disengage did not last long. She said that it caused constant fighting but "it means life!" This was, she said, the worst time in her entire married life.

The family doctor had given permission for Mr Grasso to return, part-time, to *limited* work in the store. However, he became very active, and did much more than the doctor had specified. He said he could not just "sit around and be useless." His wife learned the extent of these activities by calling his assistant, a family friend, who was sympathetic to Mrs Grasso's view of heart attack recovery. She also came by the store herself and often saw him heavily involved. This was how she found out he was smoking cigarettes again. Their son testified to the bitter arguments which followed these occasions.

Most of the fighting between the couple was over whether or not Mr Grasso would ever be healthy enough to return to full-time operation of the business. He said yes, she insisted no. An early strategy he employed was to argue that he would suffer severe personal loss if he had to sell the business and then could not find a suitable job. He claimed that because of his two heart attacks, companies would be reluctant to hire him. This would leave only jobs like grocery store clerk and messenger boy open to him. He realized that both his wife and son knew how difficult menial positions like these would be for him to accept.

The appeal to his individual needs was not persuasive, however. His wife countered that the strain of ownership, and the long hours it entailed would endanger his life, and thus bring him and the family an even greater loss.

Anthony, their son, tried to mediate this dispute. Since homecoming, he had supported his mother's approach to the care. He too insisted that his father be slow in resuming past activities, and became upset with his father's smoking, his activity, and failure to take his condition seriously. This alliance with his mother caused Anthony some ambivalent feelings. Historically, the family triad consisted of father–son versus mother. Anthony did not want to lose the close affiliation with his father. Yet, he felt obliged to oppose him when he observed his father disregarding a cautious approach (see Caplow 1968, Chapter 6).

It was Anthony who suggested that a compromise could be arranged by his becoming a partner in the business with his father. He proposed that the business be expanded with him doing the heavy work and his father retaining a less strenuous managerial role. Father would plan, son would implement. In this way, his health would be less threatened by the strain of ownership and operation. Although Mr Grasso would have preferred the sole responsibility for the store, what his son proposed took away much of Mrs Grasso's argument. He agreed to the partnership.

In principle, Mrs Grasso also agreed, although she was highly skeptical that the plan would work. While she told her husband, "I'll leave it up to you . . . Whatever you and your son decide," she played "devil's advocate" when the three of them discussed the matter, and as Mr Grasso explained, "She keeps bringing up 'roadblock' questions, 'what-if' questions." Privately she urged Anthony not to abandon his plans for college and a professional career.

Father and son's plans for expanding the business suffered a critical setback when the property adjoining their store became unavailable. Without being able to increase the volume of business, the present capacity of the business could not support the income needs of both father and son and would not be a viable career option for Anthony. The plan was abandoned.

Not surprisingly, the family crisis deepened to its lowest ebb. The extent of Mr Grasso's activities in the store brought about continuous arguing, as did his activities at home. Could he go up and down stairs? How often could he attend social gatherings? Could he take his grandchildren out to play? Ordinarily an extroverted person, Mr Grasso became uncharacteristically quiet and uncommunicative between fights. He sat silently for hours, not responding to his wife or son. When friends visited he said he sometimes went into another room by himself. He explained that his withdrawal from social activities and interaction was in response to not being able to participate fully. This angered him and he left the room rather than express his anger publicly.

Once an expanded family business was no longer a possibility, Anthony's support of his mother's position changed considerably. He became openly tolerant of his father's behavior and argued with his mother to be more tolerant and accepting. Now, mother and son argued. It was not long before Anthony began to stay away from the home. He reactivated his social life and put more time into his job. Both spouses recognized that the very existance of their marriage was threatened. It had come to this: resolve the issues or the relationship would never survive. Neither spouse seemed able to tolerate additional strain. Mr Grasso decided to put the business up for sale. He explained his decision this way:

> This was probably on my mind: the fact that we have had many, many ugly disputes about this thing [the store] and I've already made up my mind to listen to her this time, just for the sake of peace. I don't like the bickering. I think perhaps even if I were making a good living, I don't believe busting up twenty nine years of marriage is worth that.

A short time after he made this decision, his wife found a job for him – at her own place of employment. It was a position Mr Grasso found appealing and it did not require a medical examination. From this point until I stopped visiting the family, the climate steadily changed. Arguments were reduced. Mrs Grasso said that she became more tolerant of minor deviations in activity and diet, and was less thorough in scrutinizing his activities. She did not complain about his smoking as long as he did not smoke in front of her. While the nurse role remained substantial, she carried it out in a less invasive manner. In my last talk with Anthony, he told me that during the preceeding week, "We laughed together again."

Normalization and Reemergence of Role Dissensus – The Ambrosios

The "honeymoon" phase of the home care which this couple enjoyed while Mr Ambrosio was a cooperative husband–

patient deteriorated steadily as soon as he began to make progress in recovering pre-illness activities. The old conflicts over division of labor reemerged with a new intensity.

The first signs of change in approach to his patient role came when Mr Ambrosio began doing chores around the house without his wife's knowledge. She had become confident of his compliance, and began to leave the house more frequently for shopping and visiting friends. She still enjoyed running the house and expressed high satisfaction with her husband's passive role. While she did the chores, he engaged in crafts she bought him. She took it for granted that he would not deviate from the regimen she supported.

Because she was responsible for chores like shopping, which required that she leave the house, Mr Ambrosio had ample opportunity to test his endurance. He would start with relatively easy activities and gradually, but steadily, move to more demanding and to him more rewarding tasks. Many things he did, his wife never seemed to discover. But when she did and rebuked him, he responded angrily. This was a change.

There was a good deal of mutual deception in their interaction. Mrs Ambrosio believed that her husband's expectations for recovery were overly optimistic. He expected to be given permission to resume most of his normal activities within three months. Nothing in his visits to the doctor seemed to dispel this expectation. Yet, his wife revealed to me that the doctor told her he would never be able to return to a full schedule of activities, and that it would be six months before there would be any significant change in his present activities at all. She said she was afraid to tell her husband this for fear he would rebel against the regimen entirely.

In an attempt to check his activities, Mrs Ambrosio redoubled her efforts to get the chores done before he did. Prior to the illness, she had tried this and failed. She had the advantage now, because he had not yet recovered his full energy level. When she awoke one morning to find her husband already up with the breakfast made, she resolved to get up even earlier the next day. When he got up to do the dishes after dinner, she rushed to get them first. The following exchange provides another example:

ES: "Tell me, you took the garbage out because you wanted to see –?" Mr Ambrosio: "I wanted to see if I could do it." ES: "And what did you see?" Mr Ambrosio: "Nothing. I took the garbage out and I felt fine. But she is not going to let me do it . . . I know that on Wednesday night she is going to take the garbage out before I do it."

Each time that this occurred the anger and distrust deepened. I asked Mrs Ambrosio to compare the demands of the home care at this point with the way she perceived them a month earlier. She said: "Then, when he was totally dependent on me I didn't have time to think . . . the strain was physical. Now it is a different kind of strain. It is a mental strain."

The conflict reached a new level as Mr Ambrosio did more and more activity openly, without regard for his wife's protests. Telling me of his daily activities he remarked: "I'm up at first light now." I asked: "Doesn't your wife object?" He answered: "I just did it, I can't take the negative approach or nothing will get done. She screams at me. I say 'right' and go ahead and do it."

Mr Ambrosio's decision to disregard the doctors' and his wife's advice took place at the same time that he had an experience with his doctor which emphasized the medical definition of his condition as still serious enough to require absence from many normal activities. He asked his doctor whether he could take a stress test at a local hospital – a series of exercises to test the capacity of the individual to engage in arduous exercise – given by a cardiologist. Mr and Mrs Ambrosio reported that the doctor replied, "No, I don't want to go to your funeral." During this same visit Mr Ambrosio told the doctor that he had been out that morning in inclement weather. The doctor was reported to have said, "You are crazy to go out in weather like this." In spite of these warnings, Mr Ambrosio increased the pace of his activities.

By the third month of home care, Mr Ambrosio just about completely rejected his doctor's stated opinion that the heart attack still posed a significant threat. He told me: "Dr M. keeps saying 'massive heart attack.' I just look at him and say

to myself – 'I wonder if you guys really know what it is?' " He
had experienced no pain even with increasing his activities,
and was on no pain medication. He began to describe his
medical problem exclusively in terms of diabetes. He remained faithful to his diet, and regularly took his insulin.
However, he also returned to near full activity.

Mr Ambrosio steadily overcame his wife's efforts to control
the pace of his activities. As his strength increased, he
assumed more and more activity around the house. With this,
his wife's spirits plunged. When he was back involved in a full
day of activities he seemed happy. His wife told me: "He
waxed the car today. He was like a kid with an ice cream
cone." Oblivious to his wife's attempts to slow him down, he
painted part of the house, dug up the garden, moved heavy
objects, transplanted large shrubs, and made plans for spring
cleaning.

His wife once again found herself without control over his
activities. She could neither persuade nor coerce him to
reduce his activities. She realized it was only a matter of time
before he recaptured most of his household chores.

Months earlier she had looked upon the changes that had
occurred in their daily lives because of the illness as positive
ones: they enlivened her life and created a positive self image
for her. At that time she told me that her husband had learned
to have confidence in her ability to play an active household
role. Her perception was that he would henceforth divide
household responsibilities. The prospect of this gratified her
greatly. She said then, "My image has increased in my eyes
too, because a lot of things he wouldn't let me do. I think I felt
frustrated. That was why half the time I was getting involved
in so many things because I don't think he gave me credit."
During that part of the convalescence when Mr Ambrosio's
activity was limited, Mrs Ambrosio discovered that she was
capable of successfully running the home, including taking
care of her husband's needs. When he depended on her she
responded, and it satisfied her. She realized how much she
needed a significant role, and how important it was for her
that Mr Ambrosio accept her assistance and partnership.

Now, she realized that these aspirations would never be
fulfilled. At one point she said, "I want to feel that he needs

me." She never returned to her community work. Our conversations were suddenly terminated when she suffered a nervous breakdown and had to be hospitalized.

To summarize, in all the families the effort to resume normal social functioning began as a unilateral decision on the part of the husband. The way the wife responded seemed to be determined by her assessment of the costs or benefits to be derived from the loss of her nurse–surrogate function. Noticeably absent from both the decision-making process of the man, and the response of the wife was any significant input from the health care system. While each patient maintained physician contact through periodic visits which the patients themselves initiated, little or no guidance in solving the difficult problems being lived through on a daily basis was obtained. It was not unusual for a wife to accompany her husband to the doctor's office, or even be present during part of the examination. Sometimes in these meetings, the wife or the patient himself revealed that the recovery was not proceeding smoothly, that pain was accompanying activity, or that the level of activities went beyond what had been advised at the last visit. When this occurred, the physician advised the patient to be cautious and to do less than he was doing. However, these admonitions had little effect on men who perceived the regimen as depriving them of a level of activity consonent with their conceptions of an adequate quality of life. More typical, however, was that the patient asked few questions of the physician whose examination touched the physical aspects of the case solely, and whose advice for living with the ailment remained generally non-specific.

With the interpretation of general remarks such as – "Do a little more but continue taking it easy" – left up to the patient and his spouse, the management of the recovery process became highly responsive to individual and family dynamics. The physician's participation in the home care was significantly outweighed by family values and social structure.

7

Study's End

One of the difficulties in planning this study was when to end it. Like the currents created by a stone thrown into the center of a pond, heart attacks set in motion a process of change reaching the far shores of people's lives. It is an event unlikely to be forgotten, and ever to be feared. Our aim was to end when enough data had been assembled to complete a life-like portrait of what hundreds of thousands of people experience every year when a spouse or a parent is striken with heart disease.

The findings of this study need little interpretation. The struggles of these eight families are an urgent call for change in the way patients and families are treated by our health care system. We have a blind spot when it comes to helping people heal lives and relationships rent by physical illness.

Having come to the health-care establishment for help, people had things done to them and for them, but never with them. Each segment of the system had its program for healing the sick and each offered an impressive array of diagnostic and therapeutic methods. What was lacking, however, was a sense of the whole.

The system as it stands lacks a means of establishing accountability for the ultimate outcome for patients. Linkages between various stages of care need to be developed. Mechanisms for anticipating the problems that patients and those who the care system depends upon to implement goals thereafter will encounter are desperately needed.

Physical illness of the magnitude of a heart attack seriously challenges the integrity of the family's social fabric. The act of healing cannot be complete until the social and emotional bonds which the illness disrupted are themselves revitalized.

As we have seen, psychosocial injury as a consequence of physiological injury can be acute.

Emotional injury and social weakening went unaddressed at a time when professional services were most available – during hospitalization. To an extent this is understandable: patients and other family members strove to project an image of calmness in order not to complicate the extraordinarily difficult situation. The facade was all the more easy to maintain precisely because it was accepted at face value by the hospital staff. In the absence of expressions of doubt, concern, and conflict, problems remained dormant until the patient left the hospital and when they surfaced the family had to cope alone.

The analysis presented here reminds us of the significance of the family's social organization. It is the milieu into which hopes for successful recovery are made manifest. Isolated by health care professionals in the hospital as a biological phenomenon, the heart attack is a social event for patients and their families who respond to it in ways that are characteristic of their psychosocial backgrounds. Thus, the event is assimilated into the family and dealt with according to deeply held personal and group values and social norms. At home, the process of recovery from illness cannot be kept out of the mainstream of life. It both shapes the ongoing life of the family and is shaped by it. Above all, it must somehow take its place beside other individual and group priorities. As the above examples have shown, this is no easy task. The social nature of the illness is clearly evident from the fact that the recovery process was deeply affected by the family's value orientation. Moreover, it was inextricably linked with other social issues of significance to the group. People in the families realized that the way the recovery was managed would affect a host of other matters vitally important to them.

Although the aftermath of heart attack brought great trouble to many of the people we have studied, there is some reason to be optimistic that such an event may for some provide the opportunity for life enhancement. But if this is to be realized, families will have to receive far more help from health care and social services professionals than was the case for these eight families. In addition, social scientists will need to provide members of the helping professions with a frame of reference for developing creative responses to crisis.

We try to help people recover from crisis, to return to normal following illness, to avoid psychological and social maladjustment.

Actually, some of the more important changes one needs to make following a heart attack are not dissimilar to those that are triggered by other common events such as retirement. Yet the retiree finds more outlets for his creativity, more support for a lifestyle in which "breadwinning" is not the central task, than the heart attack victim who also needs to make some shifts of emphasis.

We have not been very creative as a society in the area of rehabilitating people's lives. The terms used to describe the situation of one stricken with significant illness are those that bring to mind images of deviance and disorganization, not normalcy and renewal. Our challenge is not to help people avoid catastrophe, but to help them find, in their struggle to overcome problems, the strength to make constructive and creative changes.

A Healing System

In the opening chapter we set out as our goal to explore the relationship between two systems, family and medical. The data we presented illustrate the dangers of a fragmented method of organizing health care for heart-attack victims, patients, and family members alike. The idea that the wellbeing and rehabilitation of patients is inextricably linked with the functioning of cohesive family units, or that the various levels of therapy are in fact interdependent was absent in the cases we examined in depth.

The pathway through the therapeutic process may be separated into several phases, which themselves can be subdivided. Simply put, the patient experiences a pre-admission phase, critical care phase, post critical care hospitalization, and a home care phase. During each of the phases, patients are treated in accordance with goals and normative prescriptions that make sense if each phase is examined in its own terms, irrespective of what went before or will come after. If one asks, however, how each phase of treatment prepared the patient, emotionally, to enter the next, the answer must be negative. Patients, thrust from one setting to the next, with their families following behind, gained little understanding of the essential purpose of their care or, for that matter, of the nature of their conditions. Patients were processed, not prepared.

During the earliest, prehospital stage of the crisis, when the family needed help in making connection with the health care system, the members were required to help themselves by playing an active role in initiating the therapeutic process. During hospitalization, when patients and families might have been actively seeking answers to questions and strategies for coping with impending changes in their lives, the situation was structured in such a way that they adopted a generally passive orientation. During the first weeks at home, when people were thrust into active roles in the therapeutic process, their lack of preparedness fostered self doubt, heightened fear, and led to an inappropriate passive dependency on a health-care system unprepared to give support during this period.

The physical separation of patient from family which occurred as soon as hospital care began was but one manifestation of a general lack of awareness of the need for family involvement in the care process. The family members need to be involved because, first of all, they too need support. To discharge a patient from the hospital to a home in which there is no agreement as to the essential ingredients of the care plan, or even little knowledge of diet, activity levels, and the like is to retreat from, not advance the goals of rehabilitation. In fact, the physical separation led to psychological distance for which there were no mechanisms for overcoming. Indeed, this was not identified as a problem by medical or nursing staffs.

Were there mechanisms for insuring an orderly passage through the medical care system, were the patients' families incorporated into the therapeutic process, some problems would have been avoided, or at least alleviated. An effective system for preparing people to live through the crisis induced by heart attack would bring patient, family, and providers of care together in one healing system.

Like other systems, the healing system is composed of

inter-dependent parts. Communication among the parts
which was so obviously absent in the cases we examined is the
central process upon which system coherence depends.
Patients must do more than follow staff's instructions; they
must understand the reasons for them. Staff must insure
more than behavioral compliance; they must probe for
patients feelings about these instructions and gain an awareness of their perceptions, including fears and anxieties. What
better setting than a hospital conference room for patients,
spouses, and children to talk about, even argue about, the
meaning of the illness for their future? Here there are trained
professionals to clarify issues and support the group in its
efforts to negotiate the roles each will play after hospital
discharge. These same professionals must, in turn, take the
initiative in opening a dialogue with family members. Our
data indicate a serious lack of trust in this relationship which
is the direct result of the isolated position and outsider status
of the family during hospitalization.

Fortunately, some hospitals have taken steps to strengthen
the healing system. So called "step down" units and the like
can ease the patient's transition from one mode of care to
another; social service and psychiatric staff do hold family
conferences; discharge planning is taken seriously in some
institutions. These innovations must not, however, be considered adjuncts to the core of scientific medical care. They
are the initial efforts upon which to develop a dimension of
care that is essential to the patient's full recovery from illness.

Obviously, the survival of the heart attack victim must be
the most important goal of care. However, most deaths from
heart attacks occur within hours of the attack. The patient
who reaches the coronary care unit (or, in the case of mobile
units, when coronary care facilities reach the patient) stands a
good chance of being discharged with a favorable prognosis
for eventual return to a normal, albeit somewhat modified,
lifestyle, provided that the heart attack has not been very
severe or that other life threatening pathologic conditions are
not present. The medical and nursing professions should
address the question of whether the organization of care for
patients with heart attacks needs to be shifted from its present
emphasis on survival to one that stresses social and psycholo-

gical adjustment. This would entail a sharp alteration in nursing roles, particularly in coronary care units; a development that would be consonant with current thinking in nursing and liaison psychiatry. We have made tremendous advances in knowledge about the physiology of myocardial infarction, but we still have a long way to go to understand the psychosocial dimensions of this problem. However, until the need to do so is recognized, attention will remain riveted on heart monitors; the people sitting out in the waiting area will continue to be ignored.

Self-contained systems of medical care such as the prepaid group practice, which these eight families were members of, offer advantages in the areas of cost and comprehensiveness of care. Yet their complexity poses problems for coordination and integration of services. We have seen that one such problem is the ambiguity of the role of the primary physician that the family is used to dealing with for problems not requiring hospitalization. Where conditions require multiple settings and specialized care, the familiar family doctor could provide the linkage between the family and the bureaucracy. His knowledge of both family and medical care systems places the family physician in a unique position to be the conduit of communication and the nexus of a coordinated healing system.

Based on the data provided in this study, the family physician has yet to assume this role.

The Physical Environment

Recently I visited a coronary care unit in a major medical center. I was impressed with its design which provided for patient privacy, and through light and color projected a feeling of warmth and health. However, passing by an open closet across from one of the patient modules I noticed a box marked "shrouds," a grim reminder of the tenacity of past practice.

Robert Sommer begins his book, *Personal Space: The Behavioral Basis of Design* (1969:3) with this statement: "We are now in the midst of reshaping the environment on an unprecedented scale, but we do not know what we are doing to ourselves." The emphasis on patient survival by means of high technology has in the past made moot the question of how the physical environment of the hospital affects what people learn about their conditions. Likewise, the actual design of the patient's home is often not considered in the advice given the family about the medical regimen at home. The heart patient who is told not to climb stairs but to go outside in the fresh air might forget to ask how this can be accomplished since he lives on the second floor in a two family house and must climb stairs in order to go in and out. At home, he frets about the apparent dilemma he faces.

If we want patients and others to express their doubts and concerns to professional providers of care, why do we not provide the necessary setting for intimate conversation? If we do not want people to fear their illnesses, why do we place frightening objects in hospitals' public areas? If we want people not to erect defenses against the realities of their situations why do we keep them in spaces that hide or distort what is taking place around them? Why do we not design recovery spaces for patients and families with their needs in mind? In the long run, wouldn't this be most cost-beneficial and serve the goals to which our medical care system is dedicated?

Ironically, the design of hospital space is used to control the behavior of patients and visitors. It is intended to allow medical and nursing staffs to operate efficiently without outside interference. Such things as visiting schedules and age limitations on visitors are also supposed to enhance control. Yet we observed that the control which these spacial and temporal arrangements provide is often elusive and has consequences of its own: unintended and counter productive.

Illness and the Family's Interior

During its course, the heart attack was both an external threat to family stability, and an event to be incorporated into the fabric of family life itself. Perceived as an external threat, the illness was focused upon, defended against, and reckoned with by the family members, who, we saw, closed ranks in an attempt not to be overwhelmed, singly or collectively, by the sudden, unexpected heart attack. Other problems and concerns were set aside and family members generally supported one another as they focused on the basic needs of survival, at home and in the hospital.

This situation changed shortly after the reins of responsibility for day-to-day patient care passed from hospital staff members to family members. Problems and concerns which occupied the family prior to the illness once again became important matters to the members. The illness and recovery needs of the patient represented, in one sense, an additional set of problems. Yet, these new problems cast older ones in a different light. Some became more difficult to resolve, while others seemed more amenable to resolution. In any event, the patient's situation could no longer be isolated and kept apart from the mainstream of daily living. From the point of view of family relationships, the situation was more complex than previously, and for some families, more problematic.

Managing the recovery from illness involves its incorporation into daily living. The changes which resulted had more or less significance depending upon what was at stake for the individual members. To a considerable degree, people's approach to the recovery, including how they played their roles, was influenced by the likely costs or benefits of pursuing a particular course of action. This is not to suggest that family members did not strive mightily on the patient's behalf. It is only to say that people's strategies for dealing with complex situations are guided by assessments of potential social and psychological gains and losses. We saw how critical the patients' response to illness was to several of the wives. Hoping that her life would become more satisfying once she assumed a larger share of responsibilities, Mrs Ambrosio was deeply distraught that her husband was able to resume his former habits. Mrs O'Shea, on the other hand, acknowledge the benefits that accrued to her through her husband's altered lifestyle. The tenacity with which Mr and Mrs Grasso struggled over very basic questions regarding his ability to resume full activities is testimony to the stake each had in this issue. Patients were motivated, in part, to leave the sick role behind by factors having much to do with perceived costs of living socially limited lives.

Health care professionals who may be involved with families during home-based recovery from illness may want to consider the significance of the family's social organization. Patterns such as those described in this work as convergence and divergence provide a framework for family members to organize their responses to the situation. They provide a means by which one may anticipate certain conflicts and dilemmas that the recovery process will engender for families.

The concepts, convergence and divergence, point to fundamental social processes by which members of a family build a life together. As such, it would be surprising indeed if these processes did not guide people in their quest for a balance that satisfied both the requirements of the recovery from illness and the needs for continuity in family life.

We did not find evidence that one form of family organization was superior to any other in coping abilities. What we did find was that structural factors influenced coping style. Faced with the problem of interpersonal conflict over the identification of activities that were and were not permitted under the patients' regimen at home, divergent families were able to move toward a middle ground that reflected a mode of problem solving consistent with the values we found associated with divergence. The approach to this same problem in convergent families differed; instead of seeking a middle ground, there was a tendency to assign people to specific roles, which, again, is the familiar style of handling tasks in convergent families. Both have advantages and drawbacks. Coping strategies in divergent homes have the potential for fostering earlier withdrawal of the patient from the sick role and a more rapid recovery of normal, pre-illness role functioning for other family members. However, there may also be a tendency for selecting out, and focusing upon, the positive aspects of the patient's condition and at the same time playing down his limitations as a way of avoiding interpersonal conflict. In convergent homes there seemed to be a tendency to discourage the patient from early withdrawal from the sick role and to the extent that this may be motivated by factors unrelated to the objective status of the patient's health, the rehabilitative process will be slowed. Yet, it can be argued that patients may benefit from the structure imposed by a highly differentiated division of labor during at least the early portion of home based rehabilitation. The point is that family structure makes a difference during rehabilitation and that the coping strategies employed in families are consistent with family values.

A Researcher's Postscript

In this study it has been demonstrated that qualitative research may be fruitfully pursued during a period of family crisis. Family members, although burdened by external and internal difficulties, were willing to expose themselves to the scrutiny of social science research. It is hoped that in depth studies of selected cases will appear with greater frequency and provide testable hypothesis for large-scale quantitative research.

The most difficult aspect of doing this study was maintaining sufficient distance between myself and my subjects. Emotionally, I was drawn to become more involved than my researcher's role allowed. At times, I wanted to give advice, counsel, argue, and intervene to alter some course of action the family was embarked upon. At times, too, family members tried to draw me in. What, I was asked, would I do in their place? Didn't I feel someone was right and someone was wrong? Would I try to help get their point across? Certainly I held personal opinions on these issues and I did ask myself what I would do in their place. Yet at the risk of incurring a certain amount of conscious or subconscious hostility, I tried to reinforce the unbiased perspective this study required. It almost goes without saying that to do otherwise would have not only prejudiced the study but also damaged my relationship with my subjects.

It is entirely to the credit of the people I was privileged to study that they permitted me to maintain an objective stance. It is a testimony to their desire to see their experiences benefit others who might learn from them, that it was very rare indeed that I was asked not to report something I saw, or to turn off the tape recorder during some moment of anger between people.

My one regret is that the outcome for the families was not always a happy one. My hope is that in the near future we may expend greater resources in the pursuit of a way of preventing heart attacks and in coping with them when they occur.

References

Anthony, E.J. (1970) The Mutative Impact of Serious
Mental and Physical Illness in a Patient on Family Life. In
E.J. Anthony and C. Konpennick (eds) *The Child and His
Family*. New York: Wily Interscience.
Ballweg, J.A. (1967) Resolution of Conjugal Role Adjust-
ment After Retirement. *Journal of Marriage and The
Family* 29 (2).
Bell, R. (1966) The Impact of Illness on Family Roles. In J.R.
Folta and E.S. Deck (eds) *A Sociological Framework for
Patient Care*. New York: John Wiley and Sons.
Bermann, E. (1973) Regrouping for Survival: Approaching
Dread and Their Phases of Family Interaction. *Journal of
Comparative Family Studies* 4 (1) Spring.
Bloom, S.W. (1965) Rehabilitation as an Interpersonal
Process. In M. Sussman (ed) *Sociology and Rehabilitation*.
Washington: The American Sociological Association.
Caplow, T. (1968) *Two Against One: Coalitions in Triads*.
Englewood Cliffs, N.J.: Prentice-Hall.
Cay, E.L., Vetter, N., Philip, A.E., and Dugard, P. (1972)
Psychological Reactions to a Coronary Care Unit. *Journal
of Psychosomatic Research* 16.
Coombs, R.H. and Goldman, L.J. (1973) Maintenance and
Discontinuity of Coping Mechanisms in an Intensive Care
Unit. *Social Problems* 20 (3).
Coser, R.L. (1961) Insulation from Observability and Types
of Social Conformity. *American Sociological Review* 26 (1).
Cowie, B. (1976) The Cardiac Patient's Perception of His
Heart Attack. *Social Science and Medicine* 10:87.
Croog, S.H. and Levine, S. (1977) *The Heart Patient
Recovers*. New York: Human Sciences Press.

Croog, S.H., Levine, S., and Lurie, Z. (1968) The Heart Patient and The Recovery Process: A Review of Directions of Research on Social and Psychological Factors. *Social Science and Medicine* **2** (2).

Davis, F. (1963) *Passage Through Crisis: Polio Victims and Their Families.* New York: Bobbs-Merrill.

Dominian, J. and Dobson, M. (1969) Study of Patient's Psychological Attitudes to a Coronary Care Unit. *British Medical Journal* **4**:795–98.

Enelow, A.J. and Henderson, J.B. (1974) *Applying Behavioral Science to Cardiovascular Risk: Proceedings of a Conference.* Seattle, Washington: American Heart Association, June 17–19.

Farber, B. (1964) *The Family: Organization and Interaction.* San Francisco: Chandler Publishing Co.

Finlayson, A. and McEwen, J. (1977) *Coronary Heart Disease and Patterns of Living.* New York: Prodist.

Garrity, T.F. (1973) Vocational Adjustment After First Myocardial Infarction. *Social Science and Medicine* **7**:705–17.

Goffman, E. (1961) *Asylums: Essays on the Social Situation of Mental Patients and Other Inmates.* Garden City: Doubleday.

Goode, W.J. (1963) *World Revolution and Family Patterns.* New York: The Free Press.

Hackett, T.P. and Cassem, N.H. (1969) Factors Contributing to Delay in Responding to the Signs and Symptoms of Acute Myocardial Infarction. *American Journal of Cardiology* **24** (November).

Handel, G. (ed) (1972) *The Psychosocial Interior of the Family: A Sourcebook for the Study of Whole Families.* Chicago: Aldine.

Hansen, D.A. and Hill, R. (1964) Families Under Stress. In H.T Christensen (ed) *Handbook of Marriage and the Family.* New York: Rand McNally.

Hess, R.D. and Handel, G. (1959) *Family Worlds: A Psychosocial Approach to Family Life.* Chicago: University Press.

Hicks, M.W. and Platt, M. (1970) Marital Happiness and Stability: A Review of Research in the Sixties. *Journal of Marriage and the Family* November.

Hill, R. (1958) Generic Features of Families Under Stress. *Social Casework* **39** (2–3).

Jackson, J. (1956) The Adjustment of the Family to Alcoholism. *Journal of Marriage and the Family* **18**:361–69.

Jacobson, M. and Eichhorn, R.L. (1964) How Farm Families Cope with Heart Disease: A Study of Problems and Resources. *Journal of Marriage and the Family* May.

Kasselbaum, G. and Baumann, B. (1972) Dimensions of the Sick Role in Chronic Illness. In E.G. Jaco (ed) *Patients, Physicians and Illness: A Sourcebook in Behavioral Science and Health.* New York: The Free Press.

Klein, R.F., Dean, A., Willson, L.M., and Dogdonoff, M.D. (1965) The Physician and Post-Myocardial Infarction Invalidism. *Journal of the American Medical Association* **194** (2).

Liebow, E. (1967) *Tally's Corner.* Boston: Little, Brown.

Litman, T. (1966) The Family and Physical Rehabilitation. *Journal of Chronic Diseases* **19**: 211–17.

Litwak, E. and Meyer, H.J. (1966) A Balance Theory of Coordination Between Bureaucratic Organizations and Community Primary Groups. *Administrative Science Quarterly* **11**:31–58.

McEwen, J.A. (1973) A Comparison of Some Aspects of Living Before and After Myocardial Infarction. Paper read at the Annual Meeting of the Society for Social Medicine, Southampton.

Merton, R.K. (1968) *Social Theory and Social Structure.* New York: The Free Press.

Michaels, D.R. (1971) Too Much in Need of Support to Give Any. *American Journal of Nursing* **71** (10).

Minckley, B. (1979) Myocardial Infarct Stress of Transfer Inventory: Development of a Research Tool. *Nursing Research* **28** (1).

Obier, K. and Haywood, L.J. (1972) Role of the Medical Social Worker in a Coronary Care Unit. *Social Casework* **53** (1).

Parad, H.J. and Caplan, G. (1965) A Framework for Studying Families in Crisis. In H.J. Parad (ed) *Crisis Intervention: Selected Readings.* New York: Family Service Association of American.

Parsons, T. (1951) *The Social System*. Glencoe: The Free Press.

Parsons, T. and Fox, R. (1952) Illness, Therapy and the Modern Urban American Family. *Journal of Social Issues* **13**.

Pratt, L. (1976) *Family Structure and Effective Health Behavior: The Energized Family*. Boston: Houghton Mifflin.

Rapoport, R. and Rapoport, R. (1971) *Dual Career Families*. Baltimore: Penguin.

Rodman, H. (1969) Talcott Parson's View of the Changing American Family. In J.R. Eshleman (ed) *Perspectives in Marriage and the Family*. Boston: Allyn and Bacon.

Roemer, M.I., Hetherington, R.W., Hopkins, C.E. (1972) *Health Insurance Effects: Services, Expenditures and Attitudes Under Three Types of Plans*. Ann Arbor: University of Michigan.

Rosenstock, F. and Kutner, B. (1969) Alienation and Family Crisis. In J.R. Eshleman (ed) *Perspectives in Marriage and the Family*. Boston: Allyn and Bacon.

Singer, E. (1974) Premature Social Aging: The Social–Psychological Consequences of a Chronic Illness. *Social Science and Medicine* 8:143–51.

Sommer, R. (1969) *Personal Space: The Behavioral Basis of Design*. Englewood Cliffs, N.J.: Prentice-Hall.

Spiegel, J.P. (1957) Resolution of Role Conflict Within the Family. In M. Greenblatt, D. Levenson and R. Williams (eds) *The Patient and the Mental Hospital*. New York: The Free Press.

Strauss, A. (1975) *Chronic Illness and the Quality of Life*. St. Louis: C.B. Mosby.

Szasz, T.S. and Hollender, M.H. (1956) A Contribution to the Philosophy of Medicine: The Basic Models of the Doctor–Patient Relationship. *American Medical Association: Archives of Internal Medicine*.

Thomas, W.I. (1928) *The Child In America*. New York: Knopf.

Tucker, H.M., Carson, P.H.M., Bass, N.M., Sharratt, G.P., and Stock, J.P. (1973) Results of Early Mobilization and

Discharge after Myocardial Infarction. *British Medical Journal* January 10–13.

Vreeland, R. and Ellis, G.L. (1969) Stresses on the Nurse in an Intensive Care Unit. *Journal of the American Medical Association* 208 (2).

Wax, R.H. (1971) *Doing Fieldwork: Warnings and Advice.* Chicago: University of Chicago Press.

Whyte, W.F. (1943) *Street Corner Society: The Social Structure of an Italian Slum.* Chicago: University of Chicago Press.

Williams, C.C. and Rice, D.G. (1977) The Intensive Care Unit: Social Work Intervention with Families of Critically Ill Patients. *Social Work in Health Care* 2 (4).

Subject Index

abandonment, feelings of, 79–80
activity: change in, 18, 116; describing
to physician, 66–7; family attitude
to, 42, 44–5, 59–60, 62, 76–7,
100–01, 136; and General Ward,
56–8, 59–60, 63–4, 65; on
homecoming, 74–6, 98–9, 116–17,
135–36, 161; on ICU, 47–51, 54;
and normalization, 136–61;
overdoing, 65, 67, 141–42, 148,
149–51; patient's attitude to, 45, 47,
48–51, 56–8, 65, 100–01, 136;
physician's attitude to, 147, 161;
and spatial change, 99
adaptation: family methods, 102–04,
144; convergent, 115–17, 133–34,
170; discordant, 115–23, 133;
divergent, 104–14
adjustment: uneven, 22, 135
admission: and delay, 2–6, 31; and
family, 33–5, 165; procedures, 33–7
aging: premature, 137
alienation: and role changes, 22, 103
Ambrosio case study, 26–7; activity,
50, 56–7, 61, 116, 136, 138–39,
152–54, 158–60, 169; adaptation,
115–16, 117–18; admission, 4–5;
control in, 118–19, 158–59, 160;
deception, 117, 158; diabetes, 69,
139, 160; diet, 121; and discharge,
69, 79–80; and information, 62;
marriage gains, 121, 122–23, 160;
and medical care, 130, 159;
normalization, 138, 152–54, 157–61,
169; passivity, 51–2, 57–8, 118, 121;
questioning, 51–2; roles, 86, 93–5,
96, 99, 118–19, 158–59, 169; room
used, 99; sense of urgency, 138;
symptoms, 78; transfer, 55, 57–8
angina, 107, 108, 110, 139, 140, 141,

142–43, 148
antagonism, 103; see also conflict
anxiety: change in, 18; of death, 17,
18, 32, 36, 43, 47, 60; on diagnosis,
31, 34–5; family's, 43, 74–5,
76–7, 107; help with, 162–64;
hidden, 107; on homecoming, 74–7;
patient's, 47–9; see also stress
Asti case study, 27; activity, 63–4, 66,
106, 111–12, 136–37, 140–41, 145,
147; children, 89, 90, 92, 105,
112–13, 145–46; conflict, 77, 89, 90,
112–13, 140–41, 145–46; diet, 80,
112, 146, 147; divergence, 85,
89–90, 113; family disengagement,
104, 105, 111–13; and family
physician, 72, 146–47; and General
Ward, 56, 57, 58, 63–4; home care,
111–13, 145–48; normalization,
136–37, 138, 142, 145–48;
questioning, 51, 106; symptoms, 78,
142, 145, 147; transfer, 55, 58;
uncertainty, 106, 111, 140, 145, 147;
union physician, 146–47
autonomy: patient's, 114, 115; see also
control

behavior, see activity
bureaucracy: medical, see medical
system

car: driving, 3, 5, 137
cardiologists, see specialists
case studies, 26–30; recruitment, 7–9
caution: on discharge, 74–7, 81
change: in activity, 18, 116; continual,
135; and normalization, 136
children: relations with, 123–24; see
also individual case studies
chores, see tasks

Name Index